WALL PILATES WORKOUTS
FOR BEGINNERS 2023

Improve Your Body Strength, Posture, Flexibility, and Body Awareness with a Varied and Dynamic Workout Experience.

Marcella Ida Nowell

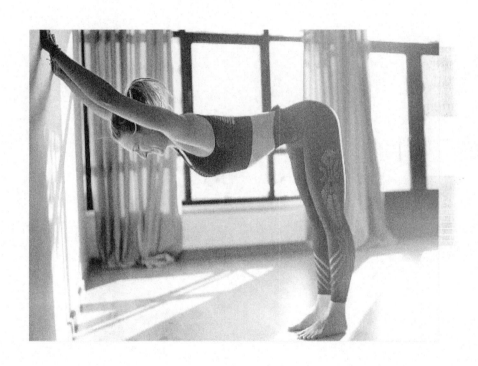

TABLE OF CONTENTS

INTRODUCTION

Pilates refers to a method of physical activity and fitness training. Its aim is to strengthen and harmonize both the physical and mental aspects. Pilates has proven significant through the systematic refinement of Pilates workouts. Not only is it beneficial for those who desire to attain or maintain optimal physical and mental health. Not only is it a crucial aid in improving athletic skills, but it also contributes significantly to physical recuperation.

The Pilates approach comprises precise exercises that are aimed at enhancing both the physical and mental aspects of an individual. These exercises are carried out on specialized mats and Pilates machines specifically designed to ensure correct execution.

Joseph Hubertus Pilates invented a unique exercise routine that focuses on both the physical and mental aspects of the body. You can transform both your physical sensations and movements by practicing Pilates. Subsequently, we will inform you of all the advantages that Pilates has to offer.

What is Pilates and what is it for?

Pilates aids in advancing both physical and mental well-being. During our Pilates sessions, we discuss the importance of achieving balance and control. Whether you are looking for beginner or advanced Pilates, it is irrelevant. Pilates contributes to the development of our muscle strength, and flexibility, and enhances our mental tranquility. Later, we will disclose to you the advantages of Pilates.

The Principles of Pilates:

- Concentration: Pilates emphasizes the significance of careful development and mental center amid each workout. By concentrating on the exact execution of developments, professionals can maximize the benefits and accomplish the ideal that comes about.
- Control: Central to Pilates is the concept of control. The works out are outlined to be performed with exactness, guaranteeing smooth and liquid developments. Controlling

the body's movement advances steadiness, coordination, and body mindfulness.

- Centering: Pilates places critical accentuation on the center, which is regularly alluded to as the "powerhouse" of the body. Centering includes locks in the profound stomach muscles, lower back, and pelvic floor to set up a solid establishment for development and back in general body arrangement.

- Breathing: Appropriate breathing methods play a vital part in Pilates. The strategy empowers profound, diaphragmatic breathing, which makes a difference oxygenate the muscles, progresses circulation and advances unwinding.

- Accuracy: Accuracy in Pilates alludes to executing each development with exactness and consideration of detail. It includes adjusting the body accurately, locking in the fitting muscles, and keeping up legitimate shape all through the workout.

- Flow: Ease and smooth moves between developments are fundamental in Pilates. The works out are implied to be performed in a nonstop, streaming way, permitting for elegant and effective development designs.

INTRODUCTION TO WALL PILATES: ENHANCING YOUR PRACTICE

Wall Pilates is a unique and innovative approach to the traditional Pilates method that utilizes a wall as a prop and source of support. This variation of Pilates offers numerous benefits, particularly for beginners who are looking to build strength, improve stability, and enhance their overall Pilates practice. In this section, we will explore the essence of Wall Pilates, its advantages, and how it can elevate your fitness journey.

UNDERSTANDING WALL PILATES

Wall Pilates involves incorporating a wall into your Pilates routine to add stability, support, and resistance to exercises. The wall acts as a guide and allows you to focus on proper alignment and form, providing a solid foundation for your movements. Pilates is a low-impact, full-body workout that focuses on developing core strength, improving flexibility, and promoting optimal body alignment. The traditional Pilates method incorporates mat-based exercises and equipment-based workouts that utilize springs and resistance to challenge the body. Wall Pilates is a variation of the traditional Pilates method that integrates a wall as a prop and support system.

- **Use of the Wall:**

The most apparent difference between Wall Pilates and traditional Pilates is the use of a wall. In Wall Pilates, the wall acts as a guide and support system, providing a stable foundation for exercises. The wall also enables practitioners to focus on proper alignment and form, ensuring that the movements are executed correctly. Traditional Pilates, on the other hand, primarily utilizes a mat or specialized equipment like the reformer, Cadillac, and chair.

- **Focus on Stability:**

Wall Pilates emphasizes stability and control, making it an ideal practice for beginners. The wall provides a solid surface for support, enabling practitioners to find balance and stability during challenging exercises. The focus on stability in Wall Pilates is crucial as it promotes proper alignment and reduces the risk of injury. Traditional Pilates also focuses on stability, but the exercises can be more challenging and require greater strength and control.

- **Enhanced Core Engagement:**

Both Wall Pilates and traditional Pilates are known for their focus on core strength. However, Wall Pilates takes it up a notch by encouraging deep activation of the core muscles. The wall provides resistance and support, enabling practitioners to engage their core muscles more effectively. This intense focus on core engagement can lead to faster and more noticeable results. Traditional Pilates also emphasizes core strength but utilizes specialized equipment to provide resistance.

- **Increased Body Awareness:**

Wall Pilates promotes body awareness by heightening the practitioner's sense of proprioception, or the awareness of their body's position in space. Practitioners become more attuned to their movements and the alignment of their body in relation to the wall. The wall acts as a visual and tactile guide, enabling practitioners to develop a better understanding of their body's movements. Traditional Pilates also promotes body awareness but may not offer the same level of feedback as the wall.

- **Versatility and Scalability:**

Wall Pilates exercises are highly versatile and scalable, making it suitable for beginners as well as experienced practitioners. The exercises can be modified to suit different fitness levels and abilities, enabling practitioners to progress at their own pace. Traditional Pilates exercises can also be modified, but the use of specialized equipment can limit their scalability.

- **Low Impact Exercise:**

Wall Pilates offers a major advantage as it is a form of exercise that is gentle on the body. Low-impact physical activities are the ones that reduce pressure on the bones and joints but still serve as stimulating exercise. Explore the mechanics of how Wall Pilates facilitates a workout that is gentle on the joints and has a reduced physical impact.

Wall Pilates exercises have been created to be tender on the joints, making them joint-friendly. The presence of a wall has a positive effect on joints that bear weight, specifically the hips, knees, and ankles, by diminishing the amount of impact and stress they experience. This makes it a perfect option for people who suffer from joint problems, or arthritis or are in the process of healing from injuries.

The possibility of getting injured is minimized through Wall Pilates due to the controlled and gradual movements it entails. By focusing on achieving correct form and posture, you can ensure that your movements are not only safe but also optimized for efficient biomechanical function. The wall serves as a stabilizer and guards fragile body parts against undue pressure.

Wall Pilates maintains a neutral spine alignment that is vital for maintaining spinal health, thereby minimizing strain on the spine. The presence of a wall helps to ensure that your spine is in proper alignment during workouts, which in turn minimizes the chances of compromising the spinal muscles or discs owing to excessive flexion or extension. It is a fitting choice for people who suffer from back problems or desire to enhance their body alignment.

Wall Pilates allows you to regulate the intensity of your exercise. The degree of resistance from the wall can be customized by altering the proximity or changing the movement angles. By utilizing this feature, you can customize your exercise routine according to your current level of fitness and incrementally raise the level of difficulty as you advance.

- **Better Alignment:**

Wall Pilates focuses greatly on attaining and preserving improved positioning during the workouts. Let's examine in more detail how Wall Pilates can enhance your alignment.

The wall functions as both a visual and physical point of reference for achieving proper alignment. This can aid in enhancing your consciousness of your physical stance and facilitate the maintenance of correct posture while performing the workouts. By applying pressure to the wall, you can enhance your comprehension of the proper positioning of your physique in the surrounding area.

The central focus of the Wall Pilates method is to engage one's core to ensure improved alignment. By engaging the deep abdominal muscles, back muscles, and pelvic floor, one can enhance stability in the spine and pelvis, resulting in a more favorable alignment. The knowledge and participation in strengthening the central muscles aid in sustaining accurate positioning throughout physical activities and everyday routines.

Several Pilates exercises on the wall concentrate on aligning and lengthening the spine. The wall promotes the elongation of the spine by offering both assistance and feedback, resulting in a gap between the vertebrae. Doing so could alleviate pressure and tightness on the spine, which may lead to better posture and enhanced wellness of the entire spinal region.

Wall Pilates improves body awareness and proprioception, both of which are essential for achieving improved alignment through enhanced muscle activation. By emphasizing accurate muscle activation and the excellence of movement, one can enhance their comprehension of appropriate bodily alignment and how it should feel. By developing such awareness, individuals can enhance their daily postures and alignments beyond the practice of Pilates.

Wall Pilates frequently includes corrective exercises aimed at addressing postural imbalances or alignment problems. These physical activities aid in correcting unevenness, discrepancies in muscle strength, and misalignment issues which enhance overall alignment and minimize the likelihood of injuries caused by inefficient posture.

IMPORTANCE OF BREATHING

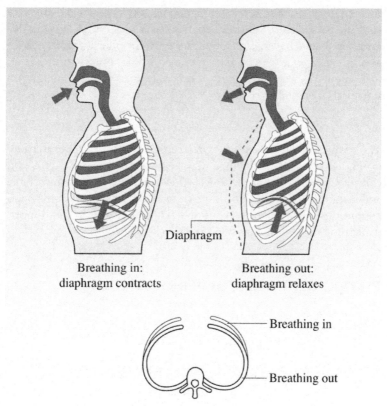

Breathing in:
diaphragm contracts

Breathing out:
diaphragm relaxes

Diaphragm

Breathing in

Breathing out

Rib pair positions during
inspiration and expiration

The act of breathing is a vital component of our being, and its significance surpasses simply supplying our physical bodies with oxygen. Having knowledge and application of correct breathing methods in exercise, Pilates can greatly boost the efficiency and advantages of the workout. Exploring the significance of proper breathing and discovering effective techniques for breathing exercises - let's delve further into this topic.

How many times a week and for how long should one engage in a breathing exercise?

1. **Frequency:**

In a perfect world, practicing breathing works out each day can abdicate the foremost critical benefits. Be that as it may, if every day hone appears challenging, pointing for at slightest three to four sessions per week can still give discernible points of interest. Consistency is key, so finding a schedule that works for you and staying to it is vital.

2. **Length:**

The term of breathing exercises can run from some minutes to more expanded sessions. Fledglings may begin with shorter lengths and continuously increment the time as they ended up more comfortable and experienced. Point for a least five minutes per session, and continuously work your way up to 10-20 minutes or indeed longer, depending on your inclinations and accessibility.

PHYSICAL BENEFITS OF BREATHING

- **Role of Oxygen in Energy Production:**

The Importance of Oxygen in Generating Energy.

The body's energy production process is heavily dependent on the presence of oxygen. The process of cellular respiration involves the use of oxygen to decompose various nutrients including glucose, which consequently results in the liberation of energy in the form of ATP.

The proper functioning of several bodily systems and activities, comprising muscle contraction, metabolism, and overall physical performance, depends crucially on this energy. Effective breathing enables the body to have sufficient levels of oxygen to meet its energy requirements.

Importance of Oxygen for Brain Function:

The brain needs a sufficient supply of oxygen to perform its functions efficiently. Although it makes up just 2% of the total body weight, the brain utilizes approximately 20% of the oxygen we breathe in. The presence of oxygen is essential for preserving the proper structure and performance of the cells in the brain. Inadequate delivery of oxygen to the brain may result in cognitive deficits, reduced attentiveness, concentration challenges, and memory glitches.

- **The elimination of carbon dioxide**

The contribution of carbon dioxide to regulating the pH level is significant.

Cellular metabolism produces a byproduct called carbon dioxide (CO_2). The buildup of carbon dioxide can cause instability in the body's pH levels, impacting multiple bodily functions. The acid-base balance is maintained through the respiratory system, as it aids in removing surplus carbon dioxide through the process of exhalation. Effective respiration plays a significant role in controlling the CO_2 levels in the blood, which aids in achieving balance in physiological functions and pH stability.

Elimination of Waste through Exhalation:

The act of respiration permits the elimination of byproducts, such as carbon dioxide, from the system. When we breathe in oxygen, the cells in our body create carbon dioxide as a result. Using the exhalation process, the lungs eliminate carbon dioxide to avoid its buildup in the system. Efficient disposal of waste substances is crucial in preserving respiratory well-being and sustaining the optimal operation of bodily organs and systems, thereby securing appropriate cellular function and stability.

HEALTH BENEFITS OF BREATHING

- **Stress Reduction:**

The initiation of the parasympathetic nervous system:

Utilizing deep and mindful breathing triggers the parasympathetic nervous system, responsible for the body's relaxation and digestion

19

response. When the parasympathetic nervous system becomes active, it opposes the actions of the sympathetic nervous system, which is responsible for the fight-or-flight reaction and encourages a feeling of soothing and tranquility. You can encourage your body to let go of stress, alleviate unease, and create feelings of calm by practicing slow and deep inhalation.

The management of cortisol levels:

The body releases cortisol as a response to stress, which is widely recognized as the stress hormone. Consistent stress and heightened levels of cortisol can cause harmful impacts on both physical and mental well-being. The act of taking slow, deep breaths is effective in regulating the levels of cortisol, as it can lower stress levels and induce a state of relaxation. Breathing techniques play a significant role in managing stress, enhancing one's state of mind, and promoting emotional stability by reducing the production of cortisol.

- **Enhanced breathing capacity:**

Enhancement of the Muscles Involved in Breathing:

The act of performing deep breathing exercises, specifically ones that involve the diaphragm, has the potential to enhance the strength and effectiveness of the muscles essential for respiration. The muscle primarily accountable for inhalation is the diaphragm, and by deliberately engaging it during profound breaths, you can boost its potency and effectiveness. Enhancing the muscles involved in respiration leads to enhanced management of breathing patterns, heightened lung capacity, and augmented ability to sustain respiratory activity.

An enhancement in the ability of the lungs to hold air:

By practicing deep breathing regularly, one can increase their lung capacity, enabling them to breathe in more oxygen during each breath. Intentionally inhaling at a leisurely pace and exhaling deeply stimulates your lungs to their fullest potential, prompting the lung tissues to expand and become more pliable. Enhanced pulmonary capacity aids in the effective exchange of oxygen and promotes respiration efficiency, delivering enough oxygen to the body for optimal performance.

- **An improved defense mechanism of the body against harmful pathogens:**

Enhanced flow of lymphatic fluids through the body:

The task of removing harmful substances such as toxins, pathogens, and waste materials from the body falls under the jurisdiction of the lymphatic system. By practicing deep breathing exercises, the lymphatic circulation can be enhanced which in turn assists with eliminating toxins and waste substances from the body tissues. Breathing techniques can boost lymphatic flow, which in turn aids in maintaining a robust immune system, thus improving the body's ability to fend off illnesses and infections. Maximizing the Immune System's Efficiency through Adequate Tissue Oxygenation.

The adequate operation of immune cells and mechanisms heavily relies on the presence of oxygen. Taking deep breaths helps tissues receive enough oxygen, which gives immune cells the necessary energy for optimal performance. Sufficient oxygenation of tissues facilitates the immune system's activities such as creating antibodies, identifying harmful microorganisms, and eradicating infected or anomalous cells.

Integrating deliberate and attentive breathing exercises into your everyday regimen can offer various health advantages such as alleviating stress, enhancing respiratory capacity, and boosting immunity. These advantages are instrumental in promoting general wellness, bodily fitness, and the ability to withstand and overcome stress and difficulties.

MENTAL AND EMOTIONAL BENEFITS OF BREATHING

- **Relaxation and Mindfulness:**

Deep Breathing Techniques for Stress Relief:

Deep breathing exercises are powerful tools for relieving stress and promoting relaxation. By engaging in deep breaths, you activate the body's relaxation response, which helps reduce the production of stress hormones and induces a sense of calm. Deep breathing allows you to slow down and take intentional, slow breaths, which can help lower heart rate, decrease blood pressure, and alleviate muscle tension. This technique is especially effective in times of heightened stress or anxiety.

Promotion of Present-Moment Awareness:

Conscious breathing practices serve as gateways to mindfulness. When you focus your attention on your breath, you bring yourself into the present moment. Mindful breathing involves observing the sensations of each breath without judgment or attachment.

This practice cultivates present-moment awareness, helping you let go of thoughts about the past or worries about the future. By grounding yourself in the present through your breath, you can experience a greater sense of calm, clarity, and connection with the present moment.

- **Improved Focus and Concentration:**

Oxygen Supply to the Brain:

Deep breathing techniques enhance the oxygen supply to the brain. When you take slow, deep breaths, your intake a larger volume of oxygen, which is essential for optimal brain function. Oxygen fuels the brain's activities, supporting cognitive processes such as memory, attention, and information processing. By ensuring a steady flow of oxygen through deep breathing, you enhance focus, mental clarity, and overall cognitive performance.

Regulation of Brainwave Patterns:

Deep breathing exercises have been found to influence brainwave patterns. They can promote an increase in alpha brainwave activity, associated with a relaxed and focused state of mind. Alpha waves are linked to improved concentration, creativity, and a sense of calm alertness.

By regulating brainwave patterns through controlled breathing, you can enhance your ability to concentrate, sustain attention, and enter a state of flow where productivity and performance are optimized.

Incorporating deep breathing exercises into your daily routine can provide significant mental and emotional benefits.

Whether you seek relaxation, stress relief, improved focus, or enhanced mindfulness, mindful breathing techniques offer practical and accessible tools to support your overall well-being. By dedicating a few minutes each day to these practices, you can experience a greater sense of calm, mental clarity, and emotional balance.

BREATHING TECHNIQUES

1. Diaphragmatic Breathing:

Diaphragmatic breathing, also known as belly breathing or deep breathing, is a technique that involves engaging the diaphragm to take deep, slow breaths. To practice diaphragmatic breathing, follow these steps:

- Find a comfortable seated position or lie down on your back.
- Place one hand on your chest and the other hand on your abdomen.
- Take a slow breath through your nose, allowing your abdomen to rise as you fill your lungs with air.
- Exhale slowly through your mouth, letting your abdomen fall as you release the air.
- Continue this pattern of deep, slow breaths, focusing on expanding your abdomen with each inhalation and allowing it to relax with each exhalation.
- Diaphragmatic breathing helps activate the relaxation response, reduces stress, and improves oxygenation throughout the body.

2. Box Breathing:

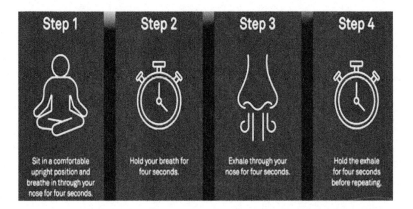

Box breathing is a technique that involves equal-length inhales, exhales, and breath retention. It is often used to promote calmness and enhance focus. Here's how to practice box breathing:

- Find a comfortable seated position and relax your body.
- Inhale slowly through your nose to a count of four, visualizing drawing the breath up.
- Hold your breath for a count of four, maintaining a relaxed state.
- Exhale slowly through your mouth to a count of four, imagining releasing the breath from the top to the bottom.
- Hold your breath for a count of four before beginning the next cycle.
- Repeat this pattern for several rounds, aiming for a relaxed and rhythmic breathing pattern.
- Box breathing helps regulate the nervous system, reduce anxiety, and improve mental clarity.

3. Alternate Nostril Breathing:

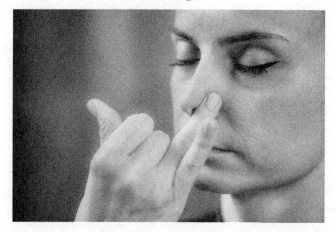

Alternate nostril breathing is a yogic breathing technique that helps balance the flow of energy in the body and promotes relaxation. Here's how to practice alternate nostril breathing:

- Find a comfortable seated position and relax your body.
- Close your right nostril with your right thumb, and inhale slowly through your left nostril.
- Close your left nostril with your ring finger, release your right nostril, and exhale slowly through your right nostril.
- Inhale through your right nostril, close it with your thumb, release your left nostril, and exhale through your left nostril.
- Continue this pattern, alternating nostrils with each inhalation and exhalation.
- Alternate nostril breathing helps harmonize the hemispheres of the brain, reduce stress, and enhance mental balance.

4. Breathe Awareness Meditation:

Breathe awareness meditation involves focusing your attention on the sensations of the breath. It cultivates mindfulness and can be practiced in various positions, such as sitting or lying down. Here's a simple breath awareness meditation technique:

- Find a comfortable position and close your eyes.
- Bring your attention to your breath, observing the natural flow of inhalation and exhalation.
- Notice the sensations of the breath entering and leaving your body—feeling the coolness of the inhale and the warmth of the exhale.
- Whenever your mind wanders, gently bring your attention back to the breath, without judgment.
- Practice this meditation for a few minutes to start, gradually increasing the duration as you become more comfortable.
- Breath awareness meditation promotes relaxation, enhances mindfulness, and improves overall well-being.

Incorporating these breathing techniques into your daily routine can contribute to optimal health and well-being. Each technique offers unique benefits, including stress reduction, enhanced focus, and relaxation. Experiment with these techniques and find the ones that resonate with you the most. Remember to practice regularly and be patient with yourself as you

WALL PILATES GUIDE FOR BEGINNERS

To start with wall Pilates as a beginner, there are a few essential items you will need to ensure a comfortable and safe practice. Let's discuss each requirement in detail:

- **Comfortable Clothing:**

Wearing flexible and breathable clothing is crucial for wall Pilates. Flexible clothing allows for a wide range of motion, enabling you to perform the exercises with ease and precision. It allows your body to move freely without restrictions, helping you achieve proper alignment and engage the right muscles.

Breathable clothing is equally important as it helps regulate your body temperature during the workout. Pilates can be a physically demanding practice, and you may build up heat and sweat.

Choosing materials such as cotton, spandex, or nylon that offer breathability can help keep you cool and comfortable throughout your session.

- **Bare Feet or Non-Slip Socks:**

When practicing wall Pilates, you have the option to go barefoot or wear non-slip socks. Let's explore the advantages of each:

Bare Feet:

Practicing wall Pilates without shoes allows for better sensory feedback and connection with the wall. When your bare feet make direct contact with the wall, you can engage the muscles in your feet more effectively.

This engagement enhances your balance, stability, and overall body awareness. Moreover, practicing barefoot allows you to utilize the natural gripping ability of your feet, which helps you maintain stability and prevent slipping during various exercises against the wall.

It also promotes the strength and flexibility of your foot muscles, which is beneficial for overall foot health.

Non-Slip Socks:

Non-slip socks are another option for wall Pilates. These socks are specifically designed with rubberized grips on the soles to provide traction and stability. They can be a good choice if you prefer having a layer of protection between your feet and the wall or if you have concerns about hygiene.

Non-slip socks offer a secure grip on the surface, reducing the risk of slipping or sliding during movements. They can be particularly useful if you are practicing on a surface that may not have the same level of grip as a wall or if you have any foot conditions that require additional support or cushioning.

- **Yoga Mat or Towel:**

Using a yoga mat or a towel is highly recommended for wall Pilates. Here's why:

Comfort and Stability:

A yoga mat or towel provides cushioning and support, ensuring your comfort during the practice. It creates a soft surface for your body to rest against the wall, preventing any discomfort that may arise from direct contact with a hard surface. The cushioning also helps protect your joints from unnecessary strain.

Additionally, a mat or towel adds stability to your practice. It acts as a non-slip surface, helping you maintain balance and preventing sliding during movements. It creates a designated area for your practice, providing visual boundaries and organization within your space.

- **Wall Space:**

To begin wall Pilates, you need a clear and sturdy wall that can support your body weight and the pressure applied during exercises. Here's what to consider:

Clear Space:

Ensure that the wall you choose is free from any obstacles or distractions that may hinder your movements. Clear the area around the wall, removing furniture or decorative items that may interfere with your range of motion. Having a clear space allows you to move freely and perform exercises without restrictions.

Sturdy Support:

Select a wall that is sturdy and capable of supporting your body weight. It should be stable and secure, ensuring your safety throughout the practice. Avoid walls that are unstable, cracked, or in poor condition. If you have any concerns about the stability of the wall, consult a professional or seek guidance from a qualified instructor.

By having comfortable clothing, either going barefoot or wearing non-slip socks, using a yoga mat or towel, and ensuring a clear and sturdy wall, you can lay the foundation for a safe and enjoyable wall Pilates practice. These essentials will help you stay comfortable, stable, and focused during your workouts, allowing you to fully experience the benefits of wall Pilates as a beginner.

GETTING STARTED WITH WALL PILATES WORKOUTS

WARMING UP WITH ROLL DOWN

Incorporating warm-up exercises is crucial for all workout regimes, including wall Pilates. Performing the roll-down workout is an effective method to elevate the temperature of your spine, elongate your muscles, and prime your physique for forthcoming movements. In this part, we will carefully analyze the roll-down exercise, highlight its advantages, suggest the ideal timing and number of sets, and advise on how frequently it ought to be incorporated into your regular Pilates wall workout.

BENEFITS OF ROLL-DOWN EXERCISE

- Encourages mobility and elasticity of the spine through mobilization and stretching techniques.
- Enhances bodily consciousness and refines body alignment.
- This exercise focuses on loosening and lengthening the hamstring, calf, and back muscles.
- Enhances the activation and fortification of the central muscles.
- Improves the ability to manage breathing and strengthens the depth of breaths taken.

Perform the Roll-Down Exercise in an Intelligent and Clever Manner

The roll-down workout entails assuming a standing position while leaning your back against a wall. The practice emphasizes the flexibility of the spine, the elongation of the muscles in the back, and the enhancement of bodily consciousness. Learn how to do the roll-down exercise with this easy-to-follow, comprehensive instructional guide.

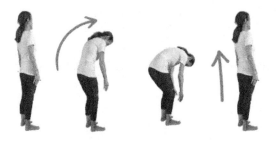

Step 1: position yourself in front of the wall, with your feet separated at the distance of your hips. Maintain a relaxed stance by keeping your knees slightly bent.

Step 2: Softly lean your whole upper back onto the wall, beginning with your shoulders and gradually moving downwards towards your tailbone. During the workout, ensure that you sustain this connection.

Step 3: To execute this next step effectively, breathe in deeply, elongate your back, and activate your abdominal muscles.

Step 4: Gradually lower yourself down by rolling your spine, focusing on each individual vertebra, while exhaling. Commence the action by inclining your chin downwards and allowing the rest of your head to proceed with the motion.

Step 4: Gradually release your upper back, middle back, and lower back from the wall as you roll downwards. Strive to achieve a fluid articulation of your spinal column while simultaneously controlling and engaging your core muscles.

Step 6: pause and take a few deep breaths once you have reached a point where you feel a pleasant stretch in your hamstrings and your hands are nearing the ground.

Step 7: Inhale deeply again, and on the exhale, start rolling back up, reversing the movement in a controlled manner. Commence the process by sequentially arranging each of your spinal bones, beginning at the lumbar region, then moving to the thoracic region, thereafter to the cervical region, and ultimately elevating your head at the very end.

Step 8: Repeat the roll-down exercise with a suggested range of 6 to 8 repetitions. The number of repetitions can be increased gradually once you feel more comfortable and flexible with the movement.

Recommended Duration and Frequency:

For the initial phase of your wall Pilates workout, try to execute the roll-down move for approximately 5-10 minutes as part of your warm-up routine. The specific time could differ based on your requirements and choices.

Including the roll-down exercise at the start of each Pilates session, is advantageous in terms of occurrence. Ensure a proper warm-up for your body, mobilizing your spine and preparing your muscles for subsequent exercises. For the best outcome, it's recommended to engage in wall Pilates exercises for a minimum of 2 to 3 weekly sessions.

WARMING UP WITH STRETCHING

Stretching is an essential component of any exercise routine, including wall Pilates. It helps improve flexibility, mobility, and muscle elasticity while reducing the risk of injury. In this section, we will guide you through a series of stretching exercises that can be performed against the wall. We will explain each exercise step by step, suggest the duration and repetitions, and provide guidance on how often to include them in your weekly wall Pilates routine.

Wall Stretching Exercises

The following stretching exercises are designed to target different muscle groups and prepare your body for the movements involved in wall Pilates. Let's explore each exercise step by step:

a) Wall Chest Stretch:

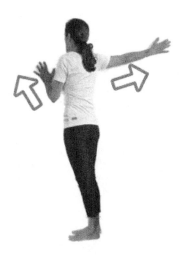

Step 1: Stand facing the wall with your feet hip-width apart. Extend your arms to the sides, placing your palms on the wall at shoulder height, with your fingers pointing backward.

Step 2: Gently lean forward, allowing your chest to move closer to the wall while keeping your arms straight. Feel the stretch across your chest and shoulders.

Step 3: Hold the stretch for 20 to 30 seconds while maintaining relaxed breathing. Repeat the stretch 2 to 3 times.

Benefits: The wall chest stretch helps release tension in the chest and shoulder muscles, improves posture, and increases the range of motion in the shoulders.

  b) **Wall Calf Stretch:**

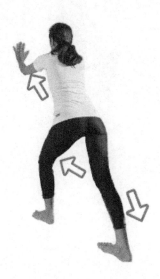

Step 1: Stand facing the wall with your hands resting on the wall for support. Place one foot forward, keeping the heel flat on the ground and the knee slightly bent. Extend the other leg straight back, keeping the heel on the ground.

Step 2: Lean forward, gently pressing your hips toward the wall while keeping your back straight. You should feel a stretch in your calf muscle of the extended leg.

Step 3: Hold the stretch for 20 to 30 seconds, then switch legs and repeat. Perform the stretch 2 to 3 times on each leg.

Benefits: The wall calf stretch targets the calf muscles, improving their flexibility and preventing tightness or discomfort during wall Pilates exercises.

c)   **Wall Hamstring Stretch:**

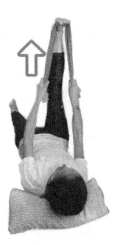

Step 1: Locate an unobstructed section of wall: Begin by identifying a wall that offers ample room for you to extend your legs with ease.

Step 2: Assume a supine position: Take a seat near the wall and recline on your back while stretching out your legs in front of you.

Step 3: Flex one knee by placing the bottom of one foot against the wall while keeping the other leg outstretched on the ground.

Step 4: Securely hold both ends of a towel and wrap it around the arch of your foot.

Step 5: Gradually lift your leg upward and commence the process of unbending your knees by softly tugging the towel towards your body, while simultaneously pushing your foot against the wall. Try to keep your leg as straight as possible while avoiding any kind of force.

Step 6: Experience the stretching sensation: As you prolong the extension of your leg, you ought to gradually perceive a mild tensing of your hamstring muscle situated on the posterior aspect of your thigh. Maintain a constant and comfortable breathing pattern as you sustain this posture for 20-30 seconds.

Step 7: Release and switch sides: Once you have maintained the stretch, let go of the tension on the towel and flex your stretched leg, positioning your foot back on the ground.

Step 8: You may perform the Wall Hamstring Stretch with a towel on both legs for 2 to 3 cycles, gradually extending the stretch duration as your flexibility develops. Feel free to repeat as much as needed.

Benefits: The wall hamstring stretch targets the hamstring muscles, improving their flexibility and length. It also helps alleviate lower back tension and supports proper pelvic alignment.

d) Wall Hip Flexor Stretch:

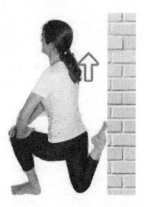

Step 1: Stand facing away from the wall and place one foot forward, bending the knee at a 90-degree angle. Extend the other leg back, keeping the knee straight and the heel on the ground.

Step 2: Lean forward slightly, shifting your weight onto the front leg. You should feel a stretch in the front of the hip of the back leg.

Step 3: Hold the stretch for 20 to 30 seconds, then switch legs and repeat. Perform the stretch 2 to 3 times on each leg.

Benefits: The wall hip flexor stretch targets the hip flexor muscles, releasing tension and improving hip mobility. It can help improve posture and alleviate lower back discomfort.

Recommended Duration and Frequency:

During the warm-up phase of your wall Pilates routine, dedicate approximately 5 to 10 minutes to perform the stretching exercises. Spend about 20 to 30 seconds on each stretch, gradually increasing the

STANDING HIP OPENER EXERCISE

The standing hip opener is a beneficial exercise in wall Pilates that targets the hip muscles, improves hip mobility, and increases flexibility. In this section, we will guide you through the step-by-step process of performing the standing hip opener exercise against the wall. We will provide recommendations for the duration, repetitions, and frequency to help you incorporate them into your weekly wall Pilates routine effectively.

Benefits:
- Increases hip flexibility and mobility.
- Stretches the hip flexors, glutes, and outer hip muscles.
- Helps relieve tension in the hips and lower back.
- Improves balance and stability.
- Promotes proper alignment and posture.

Standing Hip Opener Exercise:

The standing hip opener exercise helps release tension in the hips, stretches the hip flexors, and promotes an improved range of motion. We will analyze the exercise in a systematic manner by dividing it into individual steps.

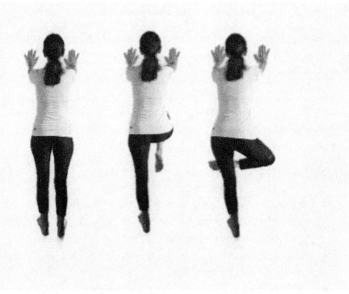

Step 1: position yourself in front of the wall, maintaining a distance between your feet that is equivalent to the width of your hips. Place your hands on the wall in a gentle manner to provide yourself with stability.

Step 2: Raise your right leg by bending your knee and placing your ankle on the upper part of your left thigh, above the knee. Make sure that your knee on the right side is facing toward the lateral direction.

Step 3: Delicately exert pressure on your right knee in a direction away from your body, causing your hip to expand. Maintain a straight and comfortable posture in your upper body.

Step 4: maintain a consistent breathing pattern and hold the stretch for a period of 20-30 seconds.

Step 5: Release the stretch and repeat the same steps with the opposite leg. Lift your left foot off the ground, place your left ankle on your right thigh, and press your left knee down and away from your body.

Step 6: Perform the standing hip opener exercise for a recommended number of 2 to 3 repetitions on each leg.

Recommended Duration and Frequency:

For the standing hip opener exercise, aim to hold each stretch for 20 to 30 seconds on each leg. Perform 2 to 3 repetitions on each leg during your wall Pilates routine.

In terms of frequency, it is beneficial to include the standing hip opener exercise at least 2 to 3 times a week. By incorporating it regularly into your routine, you allow your hips to gradually open and increase flexibility over time.

Additional Tips:

- Listen to your body and adjust the intensity of the stretch according to your comfort level. Avoid forcing the movement or experiencing pain.
- Engage your core muscles and maintain good posture throughout the exercise.
- Breathe deeply and evenly to facilitate relaxation and enhance the stretching effect.
- If you have any pre-existing hip conditions or injuries, consult with a qualified instructor or healthcare professional before performing this exercise.

In summary, the standing hip opener exercise is an effective way to improve hip flexibility, release tension, and enhance overall mobility. By following the step-by-step instructions and incorporating this exercise into your wall Pilates routine, you can experience the benefits of increased hip range of motion and improved balance. Remember to practice regularly, listen to your body, and enjoy the journey towards better hip health and overall well-being.

SIDE LEG SWING

The dynamic action of the side leg swing workout specifically focuses on toning the muscles situated on the outer portion of the thighs and hips. Assisting in the improvement of hip stability and fortifying the hip abductors, this activity also contributes to an overall increase in lower body strength. In this segment, we will walk you through the gradual process of executing the wall-side leg swing workout. Our suggestions will assist you in efficiently integrating it into your weekly wall Pilates regimen by advising you on the appropriate duration, repetitions, and frequency.

Benefits:

- Strengthens the hip abductor muscles, including the gluteus medius and minimus.
- Improves hip stability and balance.
- Increases hip joint mobility.
- Engages the core muscles for stability.
- Targets the outer thigh and hip muscles.

Side Leg Swing Exercise

The side leg swing exercise involves controlled swinging movements of the leg to engage the hip abductor muscles. Here's a detailed breakdown of the exercise:

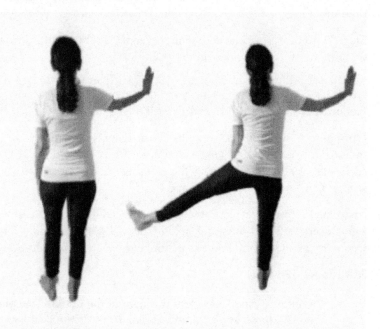

Step 1: Stand sideways with your right side facing the wall and place

your right hand lightly on the wall for support. Keep your feet hip-width apart and maintain a straight alignment from head to toe.

Step 2: Shift your weight onto your left leg, keeping a slight bend in the knee for stability.

Step 3: Engage your core muscles for stability and balance.

Step 4: Swing your right leg out to the side, leading with the heel. Keep the movement controlled and avoid swinging the leg too high or forcefully. The range of motion can vary depending on your comfort level and flexibility.

Step 5: As you swing your leg out to the side, maintain an engaged core and avoid leaning your upper body towards the wall. The movement should come from the hip joint, with minimal involvement from the upper body.

Step 6: Swing your leg back towards the starting position, maintaining control throughout the movement. Aim for a smooth, fluid motion.

Step 7: Repeat the side leg swing exercise for a recommended duration of 10 to 12 swings on each side.

Recommended Duration and Frequency:

During your wall Pilates routine, allocate approximately 5 to 10 minutes for the side leg swing exercise. Perform 10 to 12 swings on each side, gradually increasing the number of repetitions as your strength and comfort level improve.

In terms of frequency, it is recommended to include the side leg swing exercise 2 to 3 times a week in your wall Pilates routine. This frequency allows for muscle adaptation and progress over time.

Additional Tips:

- Maintain proper alignment throughout the exercise, keeping your body tall and avoiding leaning towards the wall.
- Engage your core muscles to stabilize your torso and support the movement.

- Focus on controlled and smooth swinging motions, rather than relying on momentum.
- Breathe deeply and rhythmically throughout the exercise to enhance relaxation and focus.

In summary, the side leg swing exercise is a valuable addition to your wall Pilates routine, targeting the outer hip and thigh muscles while improving stability and mobility. By following the step-by-step instructions and incorporating this exercise into your weekly routine, you can strengthen your hip abductors and enhance your overall lower body strength. Remember to start with a comfortable number of repetitions and gradually increase as you progress. Enjoy the benefits of improved hip stability and strength through regular practice of the side leg swing exercise.

SUPPORTED SEMI LUNGE

The supported semi-lunge is a foundational exercise in Pilates that targets the lower body muscles while providing support and stability. It involves a partial lunge position with the support of a wall or other sturdy surface. We will be exploring the definition of the supported semi-lunge, discussing the muscles it targets, outlining its primary benefits, and highlighting common mistakes to avoid during its execution for a better understanding of this workout.

THE PRIMARY BENEFITS OF THE SUPPORTED SEMI-LUNGE INCLUDE

- Reinforcing the quadriceps, gluteal muscles, and hamstrings, driving to make strides in lower body quality and soundness.
- Upgrading adjust and coordination through the single-leg position.
- Advancing appropriate arrangement and pose by locks in the center muscles.
- Expanding adaptability within the hip flexors and advancing solid hip joint versatility.
- Developing functional strength applicable to daily activities and sports.

Defining the Supported Semi Lunge:

The supported semi-lunge is an exercise where one leg is positioned in a lunge stance, while the back foot rests against a wall or any stable surface for support. The front leg is flexed at the knee and hip joints, creating a partial lunge position. The upper body remains upright with good posture throughout the exercise.

Muscles Targeted and Primary Benefits:

The supported semi-lunge primarily targets the following muscle groups:

- Quadriceps: The quadriceps muscles, located at the front of the thigh, are actively engaged in the front leg during the supported semi-lunge. They assist in knee extension and stability.
- Gluteal Muscles: The gluteus maximus and medius muscles, situated in the buttocks, play a significant role in stabilizing the pelvis and supporting the body's posture during exercise.
- Hamstrings: The back leg's hamstring muscles, located at the back of the thigh, are stretched, and engaged to support the lunge position and assist in maintaining balance.
- Core Muscles: The deep core muscles, including the transversus abdominis and multifidus, provide stability and help maintain proper posture during the supported semi-lunge.

Common Mistakes to Avoid:

a) To ensure the effective and safe execution of the supported semi-lunge, be mindful of the following common mistakes:
b) Leaning too far forward: Avoid leaning excessively forward from the hips, as it may strain the lower back and compromise proper alignment. Maintain an upright posture throughout the exercise.
c) Allowing the knee to extend beyond the toes: Ensure that the front knee remains aligned with the ankle and does not

extend beyond the toes. This helps protect the knee joint and maintain proper form.

d) Collapsing the core: Avoid letting the core muscles relax or collapse during the exercise. Keep the abdominal muscles engaged to support the spine and maintain stability.

e) Neglecting proper foot alignment: Pay attention to the alignment of the front foot, ensuring that it remains stable and grounded with the toes pointing forward.

f) Rushing through the movement: Perform the supported semi-lunge with control and focus on maintaining proper form. Avoid rushing or bouncing in the lunge position.

Step-by-Step Guide to the Supported Semi Lunge

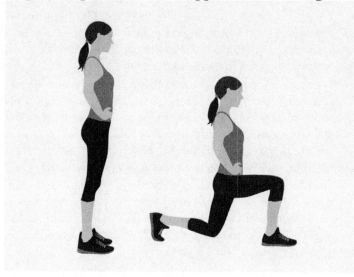

Step 1: Proper Alignment and Stance

To start the supported semi-lunge, it's essential to establish the correct alignment and stance:

- *Ideal Foot Positioning and Distance:* Begin by standing with your feet hip-width apart. Step your right foot forward, ensuring that both feet are pointing straight ahead. Maintain a comfortable distance between your feet, with the front foot approximately one to two feet in front of the other.

- *Aligning Your Knees, Hips, and Shoulders:* Check your alignment by ensuring that your knees are tracking over your toes, your hips are level, and your shoulders are stacked over your hips. Avoid excessive leaning or tilting of the upper body.
- *Maintaining a Neutral Spine:* Keep your spine neutral by engaging your core muscles. Avoid arching or rounding your lower back. Imagine a straight line extending from your head to your tailbone.

Step 2: Initiating the Movement

- Once you've established the proper alignment, it's time to initiate the movement:
- *Engaging Your Core and Activating the Glutes:* Draw your navel towards your spine to engage your core muscles. Squeeze your glutes (buttock muscles) to stabilize your hips and maintain balance throughout the exercise.
- *Breathing Techniques for Stability and Focus:* Inhale deeply through your nose, expanding your ribcage. Exhale fully through your mouth, engaging your core and providing stability during the movement. Maintain a rhythmic breathing pattern throughout the exercise.
- *Transitioning into the Supported Semi Lunge Position:* Slowly bend your knees, lowering your body towards the ground. Aim for a 90-degree angle at the front knee, ensuring that it remains aligned with your toes. The back knee can be slightly bent or hovering above the ground, depending on your comfort and fitness level.

Step 3: Executing the Supported Semi Lunge

With the correct alignment and initiation, you can now execute the supported semi lunge:

- *Maintaining Balance and Stability throughout the Movement:* Focus on distributing your weight evenly between both feet, engaging the muscles of your legs and core for stability. Avoid leaning too far forward or backward.

- *Proper Form for the Upper Body and Arms:* Keep your torso upright, with your shoulders relaxed and aligned with your hips. You can choose to place your hands on your hips, extend them forward, or place them on a wall or support for balance.
- *Progressions and Modifications for Different Fitness Levels:* Beginners can start with a shallow lunge, gradually increasing the depth and range of motion as they gain strength and flexibility. For an added challenge, you can incorporate weights or resistance bands.

Step 4: Returning to the Starting Position

- To complete the supported semi lunge exercise, follow these steps to return to the starting position:
- Push through the heel of your front foot, engaging the quadriceps and glutes of that leg.
- Extend your front leg and bring your back foot back to the starting position, aligning your feet hip-width apart.
- Repeat the exercise on the other side by stepping your left foot forward and repeating the steps outlined above.

Recommended Duration and Frequency:

During your wall Pilates routine, allocate approximately 5 to 10 minutes for the supported semi lunge exercise. Perform 10 to 12 repetitions on each leg, gradually increasing the number of repetitions as you progress and feel comfortable.

In terms of frequency, aim to include the supported semi lunge exercise 2 to 3 times a week in your wall Pilates routine. This regular practice will help strengthen your lower body muscles, improve balance, and achieve optimal results.

Additional Tips:

- Focus on maintaining proper form and alignment throughout the exercise, keeping your knees in line with your toes and your torso upright.

- Breathe deeply and rhythmically during the exercise, inhaling through your nose and exhaling through your mouth.
- Start with a shallow lunge and gradually increase the depth and range of motion as you become more comfortable and stronger.
- If you have any pre-existing knee or hip conditions, it is advisable to consult with a qualified instructor or healthcare professional before performing this exercise.

STANDING KNEE RAISE

The standing knee raise is a dynamic and effective exercise that targets the core muscles, enhances balance, and improves overall stability. This wall Pilates exercise is suitable for all fitness levels and can be easily incorporated into your workout routine. In this guide, we will provide a detailed step-by-step breakdown of the exercise, discuss its benefits, suggest the recommended time and repetitions, and offer insights on how frequently you can perform this exercise for optimal results.

BENEFITS FROM PERFORMING THE STANDING KNEE RAISE INCLUDE

1. Core Muscle Activation:

The core muscles, such as the abdominal muscles, hip flexors, and lower back muscles, are activated by performing the standing knee raise.

The spine and pelvis experience stabilization by collaborating with these muscles, leading to better posture and an overall increase in core strength.

2. Balance and Stability Enhancement:

By performing the standing knee raise, you challenge your balance and proprioception, thereby improving stability.

The exercise activates the small stabilizing muscles around the hips and knees, enhancing overall balance and coordination.

3. Hip Flexor Strength and Mobility:

The movement involved in the standing knee raise helps to strengthen and lengthen the hip flexor muscles.

This can be particularly beneficial for individuals who spend prolonged periods sitting, as it helps counteract the effects of sedentary lifestyles.

4. Leg Muscles Engagement:

While the primary focus is on the core muscles, the standing knee raise also engages the quadriceps muscles in the lifting leg.

The exercise promotes strength development in the legs and contributes to overall lower body toning.

Step-by-Step Guide to the Standing Knee Raise:

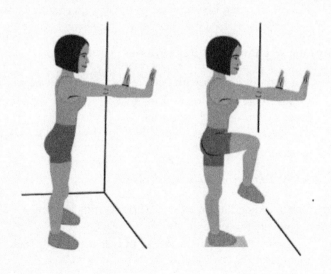

Preparation:

1. Stand tall facing a wall, ensuring that your feet are hip-width apart.

2. Place your hands lightly on the wall at chest level for support.
3. Engage your core muscles by gently drawing your belly button towards your spine.
4. Relax your shoulders and keep a straight posture.

Execution:

1. Shift your weight onto one leg while keeping the other foot in contact with the ground.
2. Slowly lift the knee of the non-supporting leg towards your chest, maintaining a controlled movement.
3. Aim to bring the knee as high as comfortably possible without straining or losing balance.
4. Focus on maintaining stability and control throughout the movement.
5. Hold the lifted position for a moment, ensuring balance and engagement of the core muscles.
6. Lower the lifted leg back down to the starting position with control.
7. Repeat the exercise on the opposite leg, alternating between legs for the desired number of repetitions.

Recommended Time and Repetitions:

- For beginners, start with 8-10 repetitions on each leg.
- Gradually raise the repetitions to 12-15 per leg as you gain greater comfort and strength.
- Execute standing knee raises for 2-3 sets in every training session.

Frequency of Performing the Exercise:

- The standing knee raise can be performed 2-3 times a week for optimal results.
- It is essential to allow your muscles adequate rest and recovery between sessions.
- As you progress, you can gradually increase the frequency or incorporate variations to challenge yourself further.

Additional Tips

1. Breathing Technique:

Inhale deeply through your nose as you prepare for the movement.

Exhale gently through your mouth as you lift your knee towards your chest.

Maintain a steady breath pattern throughout the exercise to promote relaxation and focus.

2. Core Engagement:

Prioritize core engagement by drawing your belly button towards your spine. Imagine a corset tightening around your waist to activate the deep abdominal muscles. This helps stabilize your torso and intensifies the effectiveness of the exercise.

3. Balance and Alignment:

Focus on maintaining proper balance and alignment throughout the movement. Keep your weight evenly distributed between both feet, avoiding leaning excessively to one side. Imagine a string pulling you up from the crown of your head, lengthening your spine and promoting good posture.

4. Gradual Progression:

Start with a comfortable range of motion and gradually increase the height of your knee raise as your strength improves. Listen to your body and avoid pushing beyond your limits to prevent injury. Over time, you can challenge yourself by incorporating variations, such as adding ankle weights or performing the exercise on an unstable surface. Incorporating the standing knee raise into your wall Pilates routine can have numerous benefits, including improved core strength, enhanced balance, and increased stability. By following the step-by-step guide provided in this article, you can ensure proper execution and maximize the effectiveness of the exercise. Remember to start with a comfortable number of repetitions, gradually increase the intensity, and listen to your body throughout the process. With consistent practice, you will witness improvements in core strength, stability, and overall fitness.

WALL DUMBBELL ARM RAISE

The Wall Dumbbell Arm Raise is an active Pilates workout that targets the enhancement of upper body muscles, specifically the arms, shoulders, and upper back. This exercise routine boosts muscle tone and posture as well as strengthens the upper body by making use of dumbbells and a wall for support. In this all-inclusive manual, we will furnish detailed guidance, suggest optimal time and frequency, and provide extra pointers to assist you in optimizing the advantages of this workout.

BENEFITS FROM PERFORMING THE WALL DUMBBELL ARM RAISE INCLUDE

1. Upper Body Strength:

The Wall Dumbbell Arm Raise is primarily beneficial in enhancing upper body strength. Utilizing dumbbells while working out introduces a level of resistance that pushes your muscles to their limit, resulting in the enhanced arm, shoulder, and upper back muscle strength and definition. This workout is designed to focus on the deltoids, trapezius, and rhomboid muscles, assisting in the building of a resilient and clearly defined upper body.

2. Shoulder Stability:

The Wall Dumbbell Arm Raise is a potent method to improve the stability of your shoulders. The deliberate movements of the arms help activate and enhance the muscle groups that surround the shoulder joint, which includes the muscles of the rotator cuff. Enhancing the stability of your shoulders can lower the likelihood of shoulder injuries, and at the same time, improve your shoulder's general function and mobility.

3. Posture Improvement:

Enhancement of posture can be achieved by practicing Wall Dumbbell Arm Raises. When you pick up the dumbbells and activate your shoulder and upper back muscles, you instinctively retract and depress your shoulders, which helps maintain correct spinal alignment. Over a period, performing this workout can assist in rectifying hunched shoulders and promoting an erect stance, resulting in decreased pressure on the neck and upper back.

4. Core Activation:

Although the exercise emphasizes working out the arms and shoulders, it also effectively activates the core muscles using the Wall Dumbbell Arm Raise. To achieve steadiness and equilibrium while up against the wall, it's important to engage your abs and keep a robust and secure core. Integrating this supplementary core involvement provides an additional facet of enhancing the strength of the core during the workout.

5. Versatility and Adaptability:

The Wall Dumbbell Arm Raise exercise can be adjusted to meet various levels of fitness and objectives, showcasing its versatility and adaptability. The weight of the dumbbells can be customized according to your current level of strength, and you can gradually enhance the difficulty as you make progress.

Moreover, the workout can be executed in diverse directions, which includes front, side, or angled elevations, facilitating you to focus on distinct muscle regions and bringing diversity to your physical training routine.

6. Time Efficiency:

The Wall Dumbbell Arm Raise is a highly efficient exercise for optimizing your time during workouts, making it a simple addition to your routine. One has the option to do it independently or incorporate it into a more comprehensive workout regimen that focuses on the upper body.

By targeting various muscle groups all at once, you can efficiently exercise your arms, shoulders, and upper back with a singular workout, which not only saves time but also yields beneficial results.

Step-by-Step Guide to the Wall Dumbbell Arm Raise:

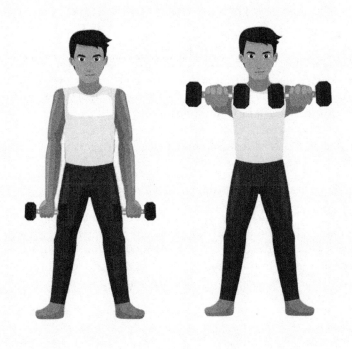

Preparation:

- Stand with your back against a wall, ensuring your feet are hip-width apart.
- Hold a dumbbell in each hand, with your arms fully extended and palms facing inward.
- Engage your core by gently drawing your belly button towards your spine.
- Relax your shoulders and maintain an upright posture.

Execution:

- Begin by exhaling and slowly raise your arms forward, keeping them parallel to the ground.

- Continue raising your arms until they reach shoulder height, maintaining control and stability throughout the movement.
- Inhale and pause briefly at the top of the movement, focusing on the engagement of your shoulder and upper back muscles.
- Exhale as you lower your arms back down to the starting position, maintaining control and resisting any temptation to let the dumbbells drop.

Recommended Time and Repetitions:

- For beginners, start with 8-10 repetitions of the exercise.
- Gradually increase the number of repetitions to 12-15 as you become more comfortable and stronger.
- Aim to perform 2-3 sets of Wall Dumbbell Arm Raises during each session.

Additional Tips

1. Choose Appropriate Dumbbell Weight:

Select a dumbbell weight that challenges your muscles but still allows you to maintain proper form throughout the exercise.

Start with lighter weights and gradually increase the weight as your strength improves.

2. Focus on Proper Form:

Keep your center locked in all through the workout to supply solidness and secure your lower back.

Keep up a slight twist in your elbows to avoid over-the-top strain on the joints.

Maintain a strategic distance from shrugging your shoulders or curving your back during the movement.

3. Breathe Control:

Breathe in profoundly through your nose as you plan for the development.

Breathe out gradually through your mouth as you lift your arms and lock in your muscles.

Keep up a controlled breathing design all through the workout to improve center and steadiness.

4. Gradual Progression:

Start with a comfortable range of motion and gradually increase the height of the arm raise as your strength and flexibility improve.

Focus on proper technique and control before advancing to higher repetitions or heavier weights.

Frequency of Performing the Exercise:

- Aim to perform the Wall Dumbbell Arm Raise exercise 2-3 times a week.
- Allow at least one day of rest between sessions to allow your muscles to recover and rebuild.
- To attain the best outcomes, it is essential to maintain consistency and practice regularly.

By adhering to the detailed guidelines and incorporating the supplementary advice outlined in this manual, you can execute the activity with the correct technique and optimize its advantages. Ensure to select suitable dumbbell sizes, give attention to maintaining proper posture and breathing technique, and gradually advance according to your own pace. By consistently and persistently working out, you can achieve boosted strength in your upper body, better alignment in your posture, and greater delineation in your muscles.

WALLS DUMBBELL ARM CIRCLES

Arm circles are a versatile and effective exercise technique that targets the muscles in the arms, shoulders, and upper back. The exercise involves making circular motions with the arms, either in a forward or backward direction. Arm circles can be performed with or without weights, and their variations provide additional challenges and benefits to your workout routine.

Walls dumbbell arm circles are a dynamic Pilates exercise that targets the muscles in your arms, shoulders, and upper back. By incorporating dumbbells into the traditional arm circles, you add resistance to the movement, challenging your muscles and enhancing their strength and tone. This exercise can be performed against a wall for stability and support, allowing you to focus on proper form and maximize the effectiveness of the workout.

BENEFITS OF INCORPORATING ARM CIRCLES INTO YOUR WORKOUT ROUTINE

1. **Increased Shoulder Mobility:** Arm circles help improve shoulder joint flexibility and range of motion, reducing the risk of injuries and enhancing overall shoulder mobility.
2. **Strengthened Upper Body Muscles:** By engaging the muscles in the arms, shoulders, and upper back, arm circles promote muscle strength and endurance.
3. **Improved Posture:** Regular practice of arm circles can help correct rounded shoulders and promote a better posture by strengthening the muscles responsible for maintaining an upright position.
4. **Enhanced Warm-Up and Cool-Down:** Arm circles serve as an excellent warm-up exercise to activate the upper body muscles before a workout. They can also be incorporated into your cool-down routine to aid in muscle recovery and relaxation.

Equipment Needed

To perform Wall DB Arm Circles, you will need the following equipment:

Dumbbells: Choose dumbbells that provide enough resistance to challenge your muscles without compromising your form. Start with lighter weights and gradually increase as your strength improves.

Wall Space: Find a clear wall with enough space to comfortably perform the exercise without any obstructions.

Step-by-Step Guide for Walls Dumbbell Arm Circles:

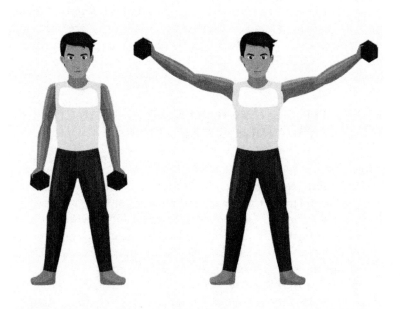

Preparation:

1. Stand facing a wall, with your feet hip-width apart and slightly away from the wall.
2. Hold a dumbbell in each hand, with your palms facing downward and your arms extended by your sides.
3. Press your back against the wall, engaging your core muscles for stability.

Arm Circles:

1. Begin the exercise by lifting your arms slightly forward, maintaining a soft bend in your elbows.
2. Initiate the movement by drawing small circles with your arms, gradually increasing the diameter of the circles.
3. Continue the arm circles in a controlled and fluid motion, ensuring that your shoulders are relaxed and engaged throughout.

Variation: Reverse Arm Circles:

- After performing forward arm circles for the desired number of repetitions, switch to reverse arm circles.
- Reverse the direction of your arm movement, drawing circles in a backward motion.
- Maintain the same level of control and engage your muscles as you did with the forward arm circles.

Repetitions and Duration:

- Start with a comfortable weight for your dumbbells, ensuring that you can maintain proper form throughout the exercise.
- Aim for 8-12 repetitions per set, gradually increasing the number of repetitions as your strength improves.
- Perform 2-3 sets of arm circles, resting for 30-60 seconds between sets.

Frequency:

Incorporate walls dumbbell arm circles into your exercise routine 2-3 times per week. Allow at least one day of rest between sessions to give your muscles time to recover and rebuild.

Additional Tips for Walls Dumbbell Arm Circles:

Focus on Form: Maintain proper posture throughout the exercise. Keep your spine aligned against the wall, engage your core muscles, and avoid any excessive arching or rounding of your back.

Gradually Increase Weight: Start with lighter dumbbells and gradually increase the weight as you build strength and endurance.

Strive for a weight that challenges your muscles without compromising your form.

Control the Movement: Concentrate on smooth and controlled arm circles, avoiding any jerking or swinging motions. This will ensure that you engage the targeted muscles effectively and minimize the risk of injury.

Breathe Properly: Inhale deeply as you prepare for the movement and exhale as you perform the arm circles. Focus on maintaining a steady and controlled breathing pattern throughout the exercise.

Incorporating wall dumbbell arm circles into your Pilates routine can enhance your upper body strength, improve shoulder stability, and promote better posture. By following the step-by-step guide, focusing on proper form, and gradually increasing the intensity, you can achieve the desired results over time. Remember to listen to your body, adjust the weight and repetitions as needed, and enjoy the benefits of this challenging and effective exercise.

CHEST OPENERS

A chest opening workout is characterized by any motion or extension that concentrates on the chest muscles, promoting expansion and providing access to the ribcage. Keeping the chest muscles limber and flexible plays a crucial role in promoting a healthy range of motion, as these muscles are prone to tighten and constrict from unhealthy posture, inactive daily routines, and specific physical exertions.

Maintaining overall health and well-being relies substantially on comprehending the crucial significance of keeping your chest unobstructed and in good health. The chest muscles are vital for many daily activities and bodily movements. They engage in activities like breathing in, flexing, exerting force, and tugging. A lack of pliability and excessive tension in the pectoral muscles can result in various problems such as suboptimal alignment of the body, restricted mobility, and disturbed respiratory rhythms.

THE BENEFITS OF PERFORMING CHEST-OPENING EXERCISES

Engaging in exercises that broaden the chest presents an array of benefits for both the physical and mental well-being of an individual. These exercises have been specifically tailored to target the muscles located in the chest, shoulders, and upper back to enhance flexibility, promote better posture, boost respiratory capacity, and augment the general strength of the upper body. Let us explore the advantages of exercises that enhance the opening of the chest in greater depth:

1. **Improved Posture:**

A lot of individuals commonly adopt a slouched shoulder and head-forward position from extensive periods of sitting or actions that encourage such posture. Muscle imbalances and misalignment of the spine may result from this. Intelligent rephrasing: To address the negative impacts, exercises aimed at expanding the chest area are beneficial as they provide a dual benefit of both stretching and reinforcing the muscle groups in the chest, shoulders, and upper back. By performing these exercises which involve expanding the chest and retracting the shoulders, one can enhance their spinal alignment, leading to better posture. Rectifying rounded shoulders not just improves one's physical outlook, but also lessens the stress on the neck, shoulders, and upper part of the back, thereby mitigating any sort of discomfort or possible harm.

2. **Increased Flexibility:**

Regularly including exercises that open the chest area in your fitness regimen improves the flexibility of your chest muscles, particularly the pectoralis major and pectoralis minor. Smartly paraphrased: Physical activities comprise actions such as widening the arms, extending over the head, and retracting the shoulders. Expanding the flexibility of these muscles can result in an extended spectrum of movement capabilities of the chest and shoulders. Having more elasticity in the chest region allows for improved functionality when completing daily tasks like grabbing items, hoisting objects, and executing upper body workouts with greater ease and effectiveness.

Additionally, it aids in averting uneven muscle development, lowers the likelihood of physical harm, and elevates athletic proficiency.

3. Enhanced Breathing Patterns:

Advanced respiratory patterns rely heavily on the involvement of chest muscles in the breathing process. If the chest muscles are tense or constricted, it may impede the ribcage's expansion, thus hindering the capacity to breathe deeply. Performing exercises that target the opening of the chest aids in the alleviation of tension within the chest muscles, ultimately enhancing the ability of the ribcage to expand more effectively while inhaling. By enhancing the lung's ability to absorb oxygen, one can experience a more profound and effective breath. Establishing correct respiratory habits not only elevates the amount of oxygen consumption but also fosters calmness, diminishes the extent of stress, and advances general physical and mental health.

4. Enhanced Upper Body:

The exercises that expand the chest not only target the stretching and broadening of the chest muscles but also involve the neighboring muscles such as the arms, shoulders, and upper back. The activation and stabilization of these muscular groups during the exercises result in enhanced toning and strength. Having well-developed pectoral muscles leads to improved stability and support in the upper body, resulting in enhanced performance when engaging in activities that require lifting, pushing, or pulling. Moreover, activities aimed at expanding the chest area usually incorporate resistance tools like dumbbells or resistance bands, which aid in enhancing muscle power and growth.

5. Relief from Tension and Discomfort:

Many individuals experience tension and discomfort in the chest, shoulders, and upper back due to factors such as poor posture, stress, or sedentary lifestyles. Chest opening exercises can provide relief by stretching and releasing tension in these areas. By elongating the chest muscles and increasing blood flow to the region, these exercises help alleviate tightness and discomfort, promoting relaxation and reducing muscle soreness.

Basic Chest Opener Exercises

Here, we will discuss some basic chest opener exercises that can be easily incorporated into your routine:

Shoulder Rolls:

- Stand with your feet hip-width apart, arms hanging naturally by your sides.
- Inhale deeply and lift your shoulders up towards your ears.
- Exhale and roll your shoulders back and down in a smooth, circular motion.
- Repeat the shoulder rolls for 10-15 repetitions, alternating between forward and backward rolls.
- Focus on maintaining a relaxed and controlled movement throughout.

Wall Stretches:

- Stand facing a wall with your feet hip-width apart.
- Place your palms flat against the wall at shoulder height, slightly wider than shoulder-width apart.
- Slowly lean your body forward, allowing your chest to move closer to the wall.
- Feel the stretch in your chest, shoulders, and upper back.
- Hold the stretch for 20-30 seconds while maintaining deep breathing.
- Slowly push yourself away from the wall and return to the starting position.
- Repeat the wall stretch for 2-3 sets, focusing on a gentle and controlled movement.

Yoga Poses for Opening the Chest

Yoga poses offer effective chest-opening benefits, combining stretches, and strengthening movements. Here are a few yoga poses specifically designed to target the chest muscles:

Cobra Pose (Bhujangasana):

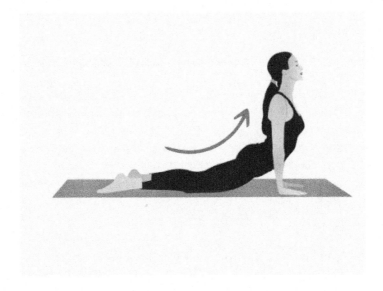

- Lie on your stomach with your legs extended and feet together.
- Place your hands on the floor, slightly below your shoulders, with your fingers pointing forward.
- Inhale and slowly lift your chest off the mat, straightening your arms.
- Keep your pelvis grounded and engage your core muscles.
- Gently roll your shoulders back and down, opening your chest.
- Hold the pose for 20-30 seconds while breathing deeply.
- Exhale and release the pose by slowly lowering your chest back down to the mat.

Camel Pose (Ustrasana):

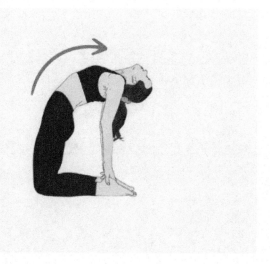

- Kneel on the floor with your knees hip-width apart.
- Place your hands on your lower back, fingers pointing downward.
- Inhale and gently press your hips forward, arching your back.
- Allow your head to fall back and continue to lift your chest upward.
- Take deep breaths and hold the pose for 20-30 seconds.
- Exhale and slowly come out of the pose by bringing your hands back to your lower back and returning to a neutral position.

Bridge Pose (Setu Bandhasana):

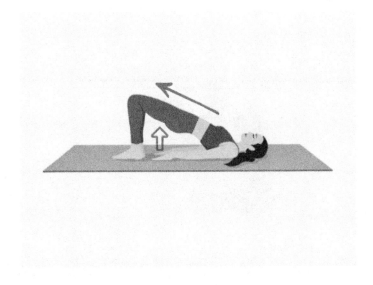

- Lie on your back with your knees bent and feet hip-width apart, flat on the floor.
- Place your arms alongside your body with your palms facing down.
- Inhale and lift your hips off the mat, pressing your feet into the floor.
- Roll your shoulders back and underneath your body, interlacing your fingers.
- Open your chest by pressing your forearms into the ground.
- Hold the pose for 20-30 seconds, focusing on deep breathing.
- Exhale and slowly lower your hips back down to the mat.

PILATES MOVEMENTS FOR CHEST OPENING:

Pilates movements can also help open the chest and improve thoracic mobility. Incorporate the following exercises into your routine:

Chest Expansion:

- Stand tall with your feet hip-width apart and your arms extended straight out in front of you, parallel to the floor.
- Inhale deeply and open your arms wide, squeezing your shoulder blades together.
- Exhale and return to the starting position.
- Repeat the movement for 10-15 repetitions, focusing on engaging the back muscles and maintaining proper posture throughout.

Scapular Mobility:

- Stand with your feet hip-width apart and your arms by your sides.
- Inhale and gently lift your shoulders up towards your ears.
- Exhale and roll your shoulders back and down, squeezing your shoulder blades together.
- Repeat the movement for 10-15 repetitions, focusing on smooth and controlled shoulder blade movements.

Arm Circles:

- Stand with your feet hip-width apart and extend your arms straight out to the sides, parallel to the floor.
- Inhale deeply and begin making small circles with your arms, moving forward.
- Gradually increase the size of the circles while maintaining proper form and control.
- After 10-15 repetitions, reverse the direction and perform the circles backward.
-

Stretching and Mobility Exercises

In addition to the basic exercises mentioned earlier, incorporating stretching and mobility exercises can further open the chest. Consider the following exercises:

Doorway Stretch:

- Stand in a doorway, placing your forearms on each side of the door frame at shoulder height.
- Step one foot forward and gently lean your body forward, feeling the stretch in your chest and shoulders.
- Hold the stretch for 20-30 seconds while maintaining deep breathing.
- Release the stretch and repeat on the other side.

Chest Fly Stretch:

- Stand with your feet hip-width apart and interlace your fingers behind your back.
- Inhale and gently lift your arms away from your body, feeling the stretch in your chest and shoulders.
- Hold the stretch for 20-30 seconds, focusing on maintaining proper alignment and relaxation.

Equipment-Assisted Chest Openers:

Incorporating equipment like foam rollers and resistance bands can enhance the effectiveness of chest opening exercises. Try the following exercises:

Foam Roller Chest Opener:

- Lie on a foam roller placed horizontally across your upper back.
- Keep your knees bent and feet flat on the floor for stability.
- Allow your arms to relax and open out to the sides, feeling the gentle stretch in your chest.
- Hold the position for 20-30 seconds, focusing on deep breathing and relaxation.

Band Pull-Apart:

- Stand with your feet hip-width apart and hold a resistance band in front of you, shoulder-width apart.
- Keep your arms straight and slowly pull the band apart, squeezing your shoulder blades together.
- Return to the starting position with control.
- Perform 10-15 repetitions, focusing on maintaining proper form and tension in the band.

Dynamic Chest Openers

Dynamic movements combining chest opening with active stretching can further enhance mobility and flexibility. Incorporate the following exercises:

Arm Swings:

- Stand with your feet hip-width apart and extend your arms out to the sides.
- Swing your arms forward and backward in a controlled motion, gradually increasing the range of motion.
- Perform 10-15 swings, focusing on maintaining fluid and smooth movements.

Chest Circles:

- Stand with your feet hip-width apart and place your hands on your chest.
- Slowly circle your hands outward, feeling the stretch and opening in your chest.
- Alter the movement of the circles in an opposing direction after they have been repeated for approximately 10 to 15 instances.
- One exercise movement to try is cross-body arm swings.
- Take a stance with your legs positioned at the distance of your hips and widen your arms straight out towards either side.
- Move your right arm in a sweeping motion towards the left side of your body, and then bring it back to its original position.

- Repeat the movement with your left arm, swaying it towards the right side across your torso.
- Execute 10 to 15 swings on either side while prioritizing the upkeep of stability and expansion of pectoral muscles.

Additional Tips:

5. **Warm-up:** It's crucial to perform a warm-up routine before engaging in physical activity, as it helps to prime the muscles for movement. To enhance blood circulation and prep the chest and shoulder muscles, engage in light aerobic activities or dynamic stretching.

6. **Proper Alignment:** Be mindful of your body's positioning while performing the exercise to ensure appropriate alignment. Ensure that your shoulders are in a relaxed position and not tensed close to your ears. Additionally, prevent the rounding of your upper back. Concentrate on keeping your spine in a neutral position and activating your core muscles to maintain stability.

7. **Gradual Progression:** If you are new to chest openers or have limited flexibility, start with smaller movements, and gradually increase the range of motion over time. Be patient with your progress and avoid pushing beyond your comfortable limits to prevent injury.

8. **Breath Awareness:** Breathing plays a crucial role in Pilates exercises. Focus on breathing deeply and fully throughout the movement. Inhale deeply to prepare, and exhale as you lean forward into the stretch. Maintain a steady and controlled breath to promote relaxation and release tension.

9. **Listen to Your Body:** Everyone's body is unique, so pay attention to any discomfort or pain during the exercise. If you experience any sharp or intense pain, stop the exercise and consult with a qualified fitness professional or healthcare provider.

Incorporating these chest opener exercises into your fitness routine can help improve posture, flexibility, and breathing patterns. Start with the basic exercises and gradually progress to more advanced movements as your body becomes accustomed to the stretches. Remember to listen to your body, perform the exercises with proper form, and adjust the intensity and frequency based on your individual fitness level and needs.

WALL SIT EXERCISE

The wall sit is a simple yet effective exercise that targets the muscles of the lower body, particularly the quadriceps, hamstrings, and glutes. It is a static exercise that involves maintaining a seated position against a wall, providing a challenging isometric workout. In this section, we will guide you through the step-by-step process of performing a wall sit, specify the recommended time and repetitions, and discuss the benefits of incorporating this exercise into your routine.

BENEFITS OF WALL SITS EXERCISE

1. **Strengthens the lower body:** Wall sits primarily target the quadriceps, hamstrings, and glutes, helping to build strength and endurance in these muscles. This exercise can enhance overall lower body stability and power.
2. **Improves core stability:** The wall sit requires you to engage your core muscles to maintain proper alignment and stability throughout the exercise. This helps strengthen the abdominal muscles and improve core stability.
3. **Enhances leg endurance:** Holding the seated position against the wall for an extended period challenges your leg muscles and improves their endurance. This can be beneficial for activities that require prolonged periods of standing or walking.
4. **Supports good posture:** Wall sits promote proper alignment of the spine and encourage good posture by engaging the muscles that support the back and pelvis. Regular practice can help combat the negative effects of prolonged sitting and poor posture.
5. **Low-impact exercise:** Wall sits are low-impact, meaning they put minimal stress on the joints. This makes them

suitable for individuals with joint issues or those recovering from injuries.

Step-by-Step Guide for Wall Sit:

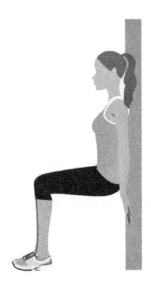

1. Locate an appropriate wall: Search for a level and robust wall with sufficient room to sit against in a comfortable manner.
2. Stand with your back against the wall: Place your back flat against the wall while keeping your feet shoulder-width apart. Position your heels at roughly 12-24 inches from the wall.
3. Gradually sink your body into a seated pose by gliding your back down the wall, flexing your knees, and reducing your physical stance until your upper legs are level with the surface. Make sure your knees are positioned right above your ankles, creating a perfect 90-degree angle.
4. To ensure stability, maintain proper alignment by keeping your core engaged and your back pressed firmly against the wall while performing the exercise. Ensure your shoulders are calm and your chest is expansive.

5. Retain the posture: Sustain the seated stance for the advised period. Those who are new to the activity can commence with a duration of 20-30 seconds and gradually extend the duration as they become more accustomed and sturdier.
6. Gradually come back to the initial stance by exerting force on your heels and utilizing your leg muscles to elevate yourself and maintain your spine in contact with the wall.

Repetitions and Frequency:

For beginners, aim to perform 2-3 sets of wall sits with 20-30 seconds of hold per set. As you progress, you can gradually increase the duration to 45-60 seconds or even longer if you feel capable. Allow yourself adequate rest between sets, typically 1-2 minutes.

How Often Should You Do Wall Sits?

Wall sits can be incorporated into your exercise routine 2-3 times per week. It is essential to give your muscles time to recover between sessions to avoid overuse or strain.

Additional Tips for Wall Sits

a) **Focus on breathing:** Maintain a steady and controlled breath throughout the exercise. Inhale deeply through your nose and exhale slowly through your mouth.
b) **Gradually increase intensity:** As you become more comfortable with wall sits, you can increase the difficulty by holding weights, such as dumbbells or kettlebells, against your chest.
c) **Listen to your body:** If you experience any pain or discomfort during wall sits, it is important to modify the exercise or stop if necessary. It's better to start with shorter holds and gradually progress as your strength improves.
d) **Combine with other exercises:** To create a well-rounded lower body workout, consider combining wall sits with other exercises such as lunges, squats, or calf raises.

WALL SQUAT PULSES EXERCISE

Performing wall squat pulses or wall squat variations, is a challenging exercise that targets your lower body muscles, particularly the quadriceps, hamstrings, and glutes. This is a stationary physical exercise that can enhance one's lower body potency, stamina, and steadiness. This section will walk you through a systematic approach to execute wall squat pulses effectively while also specifying the ideal time and repetitions. Additionally, we will delve into the advantages of including this workout in your regular routine.

BENEFITS OF WALL SQUATS EXERCISE

1. Wall squats improve the lower body by concentrating on the quadriceps, hamstrings, and glutes, augmenting their power and stamina. This workout has the potential to enhance the stability, balance, and strength of the lower part of the body in a holistic manner.
2. To perform wall squats correctly, one must engage the core muscles, such as the abdominal and back muscles, by maintaining proper posture and alignment. Enhancing core stability and posture is facilitated by this.
3. Enhances suppleness and expands the extent of movement: Wall squats entail assuming a deep squat pose, which can enhance suppleness and widen the range of movement in the hips, knees, and ankles.
4. Enhances physical endurance: The act of maintaining a squat stance while leaning on a wall prompts the muscles to endure and persist in contraction, thereby boosting physical stamina and endurance.
5. Wall squats, being a low-impact physical activity, can be considered appropriate for individuals who are facing joint problems or are in the process of recuperating from injuries. These exercises offer a challenging fitness routine without exerting too much pressure on the joints.

Step-By-Step Guide for Wall Squat Pulses Exercise:

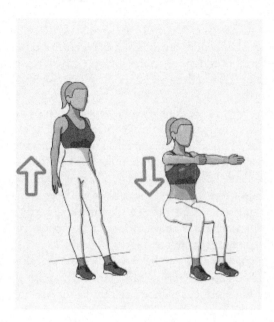

Here's how to perform squats up and down exercises against the wall:

1. Find a clear wall space: Look for a sturdy wall that provides enough space for you to perform the exercise without any obstacles.
2. Stand with your back against the wall: Position yourself facing the wall and stand with your feet slightly wider than shoulder-width apart. Your back should be pressed against the wall throughout the exercise.
3. Lower into a squat position: Slowly slide your back down the wall while bending your knees. Keep your feet flat on the floor, and make sure your knees are directly above your ankles, not extending past them. Lower yourself until your thighs are parallel to the floor, forming a 90-degree angle at the knees.
4. Perform the up and down pulses: From the lowered squat position, begin to pulse up and down. Move your body a

few inches up and down while maintaining the squat position. Focus on engaging your quadriceps and glutes to control the movement.

5. Control the pace: Control the speed of your pulses. Start with a slow and controlled movement, and if you feel comfortable and more confident, you can increase the pace. The pulses should be small, controlled movements within the squat position.

6. Repeat for desired reps or duration: Aim to perform 10 to 15 pulses as a starting point. You can gradually increase the number of pulses as you get stronger. If you prefer a timed approach, you can perform pulses for 20 to 30 seconds initially and then increase the duration as you progress.

7. Maintain proper form: Throughout the exercise, keep your back pressed against the wall, knees aligned with your ankles, and feet flat on the floor. Engage your core muscles and maintain a neutral spine.

8. Rise back up: Once you have completed the desired number of pulses or duration, push through your heels and straighten your legs to rise back up to the starting position against the wall.

9. Repeat for multiple sets: For an effective workout, aim to perform 2 to 3 sets of squats up and down against the wall. Take short breaks between sets to allow your muscles to recover.

10. Remember to listen to your body and stop if you experience any pain or discomfort.

Repetitions and Frequency:

For beginners, aim to perform 2-3 sets of wall squats with 20-30 seconds of hold per set. As you progress, you can increase the duration to 45-60 seconds or longer. Allow yourself adequate rest between sets, typically 1-2 minutes.

How Often Should You Do Wall Squats?

Wall squats can be incorporated into your exercise routine 2-3 times per week. It is important to listen to your body and allow for proper rest and recovery between sessions. Remember, quality of form and engagement is more important than quantity.

Additional Tips for Wall Squats:

a) **Focus on breathing:** Maintain a steady and controlled breath throughout the exercise. Inhale deeply through your nose during the descent and exhale through your mouth as you rise back up.

b) **Keep your weight centered:** Distribute your weight evenly on both feet to avoid leaning forward or backward. This helps maintain proper alignment and prevents strain on the knees.

c) **Gradually increase intensity:** As you become more comfortable with wall squats, you can add variations or increase the difficulty by holding light dumbbells or adding a mini band around your thighs to engage additional muscles.

d) **Listen to your body:** If you experience any pain or discomfort, modify the exercise, or stop if necessary. It's important to work within your comfort and capability levels.

WALL PUSH-UP EXERCISE

This workout routine is particularly beneficial for individuals who are new to fitness or have limited upper body endurance, as it minimizes the strain on the wrists and shoulders while also reducing resistance. This section will offer a thorough tutorial on the proper way to execute wall push-ups, including the optimal duration and number of repetitions. Additionally, we will explore how often this exercise should be included in your regular workout regimen.

BENEFITS OF WALL PUSH-UPS EXERCISE

1. **Builds upper body strength:** Wall push-ups target the muscles of the chest, shoulders, and triceps, helping to develop strength and definition in the upper body.

2. **Improves core stability:** Engaging the core muscles during wall push-ups helps improve stability and support for the spine, promoting better posture and overall core strength.

3. **Suitable for all fitness levels:** Wall push-ups are highly adaptable and can be modified to suit different fitness levels.

They provide a starting point for beginners to build strength before progressing to more challenging variations.

4. **Reduces strain on the wrists and shoulders:** The vertical positioning of the body in wall push-ups alleviates the pressure on the wrists and shoulders compared to traditional push-ups performed on the ground.

5. **Enhances functional strength:** As a compound exercise, wall push-ups engage multiple muscle groups, mimicking real-life pushing movements and improving overall functional strength.

Step-by-Step Guide for Wall Push-Ups

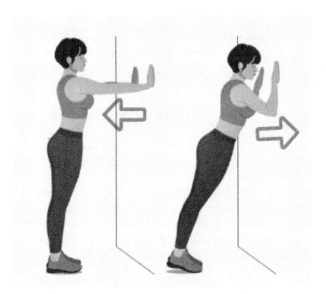

1. Find a suitable wall: Look for a flat and sturdy wall with enough space to perform the exercise comfortably. Make sure there are no hindrances or obstructions that could impede your ability to move.

2. Get in front of the wall: Stand at a distance of a few feet from the wall and make sure that you are facing it. For better stability, it is recommended that you position your feet at a distance equal to the width of your hips, while also allowing your toes to point slightly outwards.

3. For this activity, position yourself facing a wall and stretch out your arms until they are straight. Next, place your hands at the same height as your shoulders on the wall. When assuming the correct position, your hands are to be positioned a little bit more distant than the breadth of your shoulders, with your fingers directed towards the upward direction.
4. Adjust your posture by leaning towards the wall and applying pressure with your palms while keeping your core muscles engaged to ensure balance. It is essential to maintain a straight alignment of your body, with the head and toes in line.
5. Gradually bring your body closer to the wall by flexing your elbows and moving your chest downwards. Maintain a straight posture and steer clear of any bending or curving of your spine. When you go down, your elbows should be slightly facing outwards.
6. Push back to the starting position: Press through your palms and straighten your arms to push your body away from the wall, returning to the starting position.

Repetitions and Time:

For beginners, aim to perform 2-3 sets of wall push-ups with 8-12 repetitions per set. As you gain strength and improve your form, you can increase the repetitions or sets to continue challenging yourself. Allow for adequate rest between sets, typically 1-2 minutes.

Frequency of Wall Push-Ups:

Wall push-ups can be included in your exercise routine 2-3 times per week. It is important to have at least one day of rest between sessions to allow your muscles to recover and adapt. As you progress, you can increase the frequency or intensity of the exercise based on your individual fitness goals.

Additional Tips for Wall Push-Ups

a) **Focus on proper form:** Maintain a straight line from head to toe throughout the exercise. Avoid arching or rounding your back, and keep your core engaged for stability.

b) **Gradually increase difficulty:** As you become comfortable with wall push-ups, you can progress to more challenging variations, such as incline push-ups on a lower surface or eventually progressing to standard push-ups on the ground.

c) **Breathe properly:** Inhale as you lower your body towards the wall and exhale as you push back to the starting position. Focus on maintaining a controlled and steady breathing pattern throughout the exercise.

d) **Listen to your body:** If you experience any pain or discomfort during wall push-ups, modify the exercise or consult a fitness professional for guidance. It's important to work within your limits and avoid overexertion.

WALL PLANK

The wall plank is a variation of the conventional plank workout, designed to focus on the core muscles, arms, and shoulders. Utilizing a wall as a prop, one can perform a demanding yet highly effective workout. This section outlines a comprehensive strategy for executing the wall plank exercise, complete with clear instructions and appropriate set and rep recommendations. Additionally, we will explore how often this workout should be integrated into your fitness regimen.

BENEFITS OF WALL PLANKS

1. **Core strength and stability:** Wall planks engage the deep abdominal muscles, including the transversus abdominis, helping to strengthen the core and improve stability.

2. **Shoulder and arm strength:** Holding the wall plank position activates the muscles in the shoulders, arms, and upper back, promoting strength and endurance in these areas.

3. **Improved posture:** Wall planks encourage proper alignment of the spine, which can help improve posture and reduce the risk of back pain and postural imbalances.

4. **Total body engagement:** While primarily targeting the core, wall planks also engage the muscles in the legs, glutes, and chest, providing a comprehensive full-body workout.
5. **Balance and coordination:** The wall plank challenges your balance and coordination, as you must maintain stability while holding the position.

Step-by-Step Guide for Wall Plank

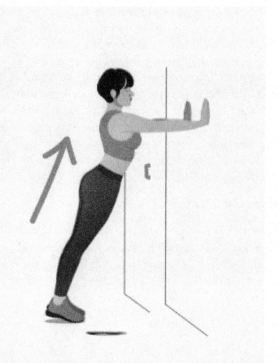

1. **Locate an appropriate wall:** Search for a level and robust surface with ample room to carry out the workout with ease. Make sure that there are no hindrances or obstructions that can impede your mobility.
2. **Get in front of the wall:** Place yourself at a distance from the wall and direct your gaze towards it. For improved steadiness, your toes may be turned out slightly while maintaining a hip-width distance between your feet.
3. **Position yourself by putting your hands on the wall:** Stretch your arms out straight ahead and rest your palms on

the wall, maintaining shoulder width between them. Direct your fingers upward.

4. **Step back and position your body:** take a step backwards while ensuring that your arms remain stretched out and your palms are pushed against the wall. Your frame must be aligned diagonally, from your head to your heels, while keeping your core muscles contracted and shoulders positioned directly above your wrists.

5. **Maintain proper alignment:** Keep your head aligned and in a neutral position, with your eyes directed slightly downward. Maintain a neutral spine position by refraining from arching or sagging your back and contract your core muscles from start to finish while performing the exercise.

6. **Hold the position:** Hold the wall plank position for the desired amount of time. Start with 20-30 seconds and gradually increase the duration as you gain strength and endurance.

7. **Release and rest:** Gently lower your body and rest for a short period before repeating the exercise.

Repetitions and Time:

For beginners, aim to perform 2-3 sets of wall planks, holding each repetition for 20-30 seconds. As you progress and become more comfortable with the exercise, you can increase the duration to 40-60 seconds per set. Allow for adequate rest between sets, typically 1-2 minutes.

Frequency of Wall Planks:

Wall planks can be incorporated into your exercise routine 2-3 times per week. It is important to have at least one day of rest between sessions to allow your muscles to recover and adapt. As you become stronger and more proficient, you can increase the frequency or duration of the exercise based on your individual fitness goals.

Additional Tips for Wall Planks

a) **Focus on proper form:** Maintain a straight line from head to heels throughout the exercise. Avoid sagging or raising your hips and keep your core engaged for stability.

b) **Gradually increase difficulty:** As you become comfortable with wall planks, you can progress to more challenging variations, such as lifting one leg or one arm off the wall while maintaining the plank position.

c) **Breathe properly:** Remember to breathe deeply and evenly during the exercise. Inhale through your nose and exhale through your mouth, maintaining a relaxed breathing pattern.

d) **Listen to your body:** If you experience any pain or discomfort, adjust your positioning or consult a fitness professional for guidance. It's important to perform the exercise within your comfort level and avoid overexertion.

By incorporating wall planks into your exercise routine, you can strengthen your core, improve upper body strength, enhance posture, and develop overall body stability. Remember to start gradually, focus on proper form, and gradually increase the intensity and duration of the exercise as you progress.

WALL LEG LIFTS EXERCISE

Wall leg lifts are Pilates exercise that targets the core, hips, and leg muscles. They are performed with the support of a wall, providing stability and control throughout the movement. In this section, we will provide a detailed guide on how to perform wall leg lifts, highlight common mistakes to avoid, and offer modifications for beginners.

Step-by-Step Instructions for Wall Leg Lifts

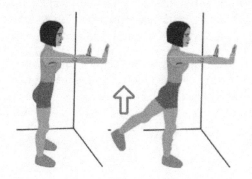

1. **Find a suitable wall:** Look for a clear wall space where you have enough room to extend your legs fully without obstruction.
2. **Stand facing the wall:** Position yourself a few feet away from the wall, facing it. Place your hands on the wall at shoulder height for support.
3. **Engage your core:** Activate your core muscles by drawing your navel towards your spine. This will help stabilize your body throughout the exercise.
4. **Lean against the wall:** Lean your upper body against the wall, keeping your hands firmly placed on the wall for support. Your feet should be hip width apart, and your toes can be slightly turned out.
5. **Extend one leg backward:** Slowly lift one leg off the ground and extend it straight behind you. Keep your leg engaged and lengthen through your heel.
6. **Lift your leg upward:** Initiate the movement by lifting your extended leg upward while keeping it straight. Lift it as high as you can comfortably go without compromising your form.
7. **Lower your leg:** Gradually lower your leg back down to the starting position with control and without touching the floor.
8. **Repeat with the other leg:** Perform the same movement with the opposite leg, lifting and lowering it in a controlled manner.

Repetitions and sets: Start with 8-10 repetitions per leg and gradually increase as you build strength and endurance. Aim for 2-3 sets.

Common Mistakes to Avoid:

Arching your lower back: Maintain a neutral spine throughout the exercise. Avoid arching your lower back or allowing it to sag. Engage your core to stabilize your pelvis and maintain proper alignment.

Lifting your leg too high: While it's important to challenge yourself, avoid lifting your leg higher than your hip level, as this can strain your lower back and compromise your form. Focus on controlled movements within a comfortable range of motion.

Using momentum: Ensure that you lift and lower your leg using controlled muscle contractions rather than relying on momentum. This will maximize the effectiveness of the exercise and prevent injury.

Modifications for Beginners:

Reduced range of motion: If you're new to wall leg lifts, start by lifting your leg to a comfortable height that allows you to maintain proper form. Gradually increase the height as your strength and flexibility improve.

Bent knee option: To make this exercise easier if you find it difficult to fully straighten your leg, you can choose to keep your knee slightly bent during the movement. By implementing this alteration, you can decrease the strain on your hamstrings and concentrate on actively involving your core and hip muscles.

Wall-assisted leg lifts: To enhance stability, wall-assisted leg lifts can be performed by exerting some of your body weight on the wall through the contact of your hands. Novices can retain their equilibrium and manage the exercise effectively through this alteration.

With careful adherence to these systematic guidelines, sidestepping frequent errors, and adopting simplified routines for novices, you can proficiently execute wall leg lifts. It is important to keep proper posture, activate your abdominal muscles, and advance at a pace suitable for your individual level. Consistent training and steady progressions in the number of repetitions and sets will enhance your power, balance, and overall ability to manipulate your lower body.

COOL-DOWN EXERCISES IN WALL PILATES

After a challenging wall Pilates workout, it's essential to allow your body to gradually transition from an intense state to a state of rest and recovery. A proper cool-down routine can help reduce muscle soreness, promote flexibility, and improve overall well-being. Below is a step-by-step guide for a cool-down session:

Wall Shoulder Stretch

1. Stand facing a wall with your feet hip-width apart.
2. Place both hands on the wall at shoulder height, slightly wider than shoulder-width apart.
3. Lean forward, allowing your chest to come closer to the wall while keeping your arms straight.
4. Feel the stretch in your shoulders and upper back.
5. Hold the stretch for 30 seconds and repeat 2-3 times.

Wall Chest Opener

1. Stand sideways to a wall, with your arm extended and your palm resting against the wall at shoulder height.
2. Slowly rotate your body away from the wall, feeling a stretch in your chest.
3. Keep your spine tall and avoid any discomfort or pain.
4. Hold the stretch for 30 seconds on each side and repeat 2-3 times.

Wall Calf Stretch

1. Stand facing the wall, about an arm's length away.
2. Place both hands on the wall at shoulder height for support.
3. Take a step back with one foot, keeping the heel on the ground and the leg straight.
4. Lean forward, feeling the stretch in your calf muscle.
5. Hold the stretch for 30 seconds on each leg and repeat 2-3 times.

Wall Hamstring Stretch

1. Assume a seated position on the ground while maintaining contact between your back and the wall and stretching out your legs in front of you.
2. Scoot your hips closer to the wall and extend one leg upward, resting the heel against the wall.
3. Keep your back and other leg pressed against the floor.
4. Gently lean forward, feeling the stretch in the back of your thigh (hamstring).
5. Hold the stretch for 30 seconds on each leg and repeat 2-3 times.

Wall Child's Pose

1. Stand facing the wall, about an arm's length away.
2. Place both hands on the wall, shoulder-width apart, and lean forward, bending at the hips.
3. Allow your forehead and chest to come close to the wall, while your arms stay extended.
4. Relax your whole body and breathe deeply.
5. Hold the pose for 1-2 minutes, focusing on your breath.

It is recommended to perform this cool-down routine after each wall Pilates session. Aim to include at least 10 minutes of cool-down exercises. Listen to your body and adjust the intensity and duration as needed. Cooling down helps your body transition back to its normal state and promotes optimal recovery.

WALL PILATES - 30-DAY PROGRAM

A 30-day Wall Pilates program is an excellent way to improve strength, flexibility, and overall fitness. By following a structured program, you can experience gradual progress and noticeable changes in your body. Here is a comprehensive 30-day Wall Pilates program that covers warm-up, workout, cool-down, and rest days.

Week 1: Foundation Building

Day 1:

a) Warm-up: Perform 5 minutes of dynamic stretching, including arm circles, leg swings, and trunk rotations.
b) Workout: Complete 2 sets of 10 repetitions for each exercise:
c) Wall Squats: Stand against the wall with your feet hip-width apart, lower into a squat position, and then push back up.
d) Wall Push-Ups: Place your hands on the wall at shoulder height, slightly wider than shoulder-width apart. Bend your elbows and lower your chest toward the wall, then push back up.
e) Wall Leg Lifts: Stand facing the wall with your hands on the wall for support. Lift one leg straight back, keeping it parallel to the floor, and then lower. Repeat with the other leg.
f) Cool-down: Perform static stretches for your major muscle groups, holding each stretch for 20-30 seconds.

Day 2:

- Rest day: Allow your body time to recover.

Day 3:

a) Warm-up: Repeat the warm-up routine from Day 1.
b) Workout: Increase the intensity by completing 3 sets of 12 repetitions for each exercise. Maintain proper form and engage your core throughout the movements.

c) Cool-down: Perform static stretches, focusing on the muscles worked during the workout.

Day 4:

- Rest day: Give your body a day off to rest and recover.

Day 5:

a) Warm-up: Repeat the warm-up routine from Day 1.
b) Workout: Challenge yourself by performing 3 sets of 15 repetitions for each exercise. Concentrate on maintaining proper form and engaging the targeted muscles.
c) Cool-down: Perform static stretches, paying attention to the muscles used during the workout.

Day 6 and 7:

- Rest days: Allow your body to rest and recover from the week's workouts.

Week 2: Progression and Challenge
Day 8-14:

- Follow the same structure as Week 1 but increase the difficulty of the exercises. Introduce variations or progressions to further challenge your body. Aim for 3 sets of 15 repetitions for each exercise.

Week 3: Strength and Endurance
Day 15-21:

- Maintain the same exercises from Week 2 but increase the resistance or intensity. Incorporate resistance bands or light weights to add resistance. Perform 3 sets of 20 repetitions for each exercise to build strength and endurance.

Week 4: Mastery and Refinement

Day 22-28:

- Focus on mastering the exercises and refining your technique. Increase the duration of holds or repetitions. Challenge yourself with advanced variations or progressions. Aim for 4 sets of 15-20 repetitions for each exercise.

Week 5: Maintenance and Reflection

Day 29-30:

- Reduce the intensity and volume of the workouts to allow for recovery. Perform 2-3 sets of 10-12 repetitions for each exercise. Use these days to reflect on your progress and celebrate your achievements.

Additional Considerations

- **Hydration:** Drink plenty of water throughout your workouts to stay hydrated and support optimal performance.
- **Nutrition:** Fuel your body with a balanced diet consisting of whole foods, including fruits, vegetables, nuts, seeds, and sprouts. Aim for a ratio of 60% raw and 40% cooked foods.
- **Rest and Recovery:** Listen to your body and give yourself rest days to allow for proper recovery and prevent overtraining.
- **Modifications:** If any exercises cause discomfort or pain, modify them, or seek guidance from a certified Pilates instructor to ensure proper execution.

CONCLUSION

Wall Pilates Workouts for Beginners 2023 is a comprehensive and invaluable resource for individuals looking to embark on their Pilates journey. This book provides an extensive collection of wall-based Pilates exercises specifically designed for beginners, making it accessible and suitable for individuals of all fitness levels.

The book begins by introducing the concept of Wall Pilates, explaining its benefits, and highlighting the unique advantages it offers. It then guides readers through various exercises step by step, providing clear instructions, recommended time, repetitions, and proper form for each exercise. The inclusion of detailed explanations ensures that beginners can understand and perform the exercises correctly, maximizing their effectiveness while minimizing the risk of injury.

Throughout the book, the author emphasizes the importance of warm-up and cool-down routines, proper body alignment, and choosing the right wall for exercises. This attention to detail ensures that readers not only learn the exercises but also develop a strong foundation in Pilates principles, promoting safe and effective practice.

Moreover, "Wall Pilates Workouts for Beginners 2023" surpasses mere physical activities. This resource provides extra insights and things to think about, including adjustments for those new to the activity, helpful advice on diet, and the significance of allowing time for recuperation. These observations offer a comprehensive method to staying fit, giving readers the ability to make knowledgeable choices regarding their complete health.

What distinguishes this book from others is its emphasis on growth and flexibility. Novices can easily customize the exercises to their specific requirements and inclinations as they strengthen their physical abilities and self-assurance. By incorporating 30-day programs, the book's worth is elevated as it presents a well-planned and attainable framework for individuals embarking on their Pilates voyage.

By incorporating wall-based exercises, this book brings a unique twist to traditional Pilates, amplifying the benefits and opening new possibilities for beginners. The author's expertise and passion for Pilates shine through, making the content engaging, informative, and inspiring.

"Wall Pilates Workouts for Beginners 2023" serves as a trusted companion, guiding readers on their path to improved strength, flexibility, and overall well-being. Whether you are completely new to Pilates or seeking a fresh approach to your fitness routine, this book is an essential tool that will empower you to embark on your journey with confidence.

Invest in your health and embrace the transformative power of Pilates with "Wall Pilates Workouts for Beginners 2023." Discover the joy of movement, the strength of your body, and the limitless possibilities that lie ahead. Get ready to experience the incredible benefits of wall-based Pilates and unlock your full potential.

FREQUENTLY ASKED QUESTIONS

1. What Is Wall Pilates?

Wall Pilates is a form of Pilates exercise that utilizes a wall as a supportive prop during the workout. It involves performing various Pilates exercises while leaning against or pressing against the wall for stability, support, and added resistance. This approach allows for enhanced body awareness, improved alignment, and increased challenge in targeting specific muscle groups.

2. Is Wall Pilates Effective?

Yes, Wall Pilates is an effective form of exercise. It offers numerous benefits, including improved core strength, enhanced flexibility, increased stability, and better posture. By using the wall as a prop, individuals can engage their muscles more effectively, deepen their mind-body connection, and experience greater overall body control and awareness.

3. Does Pilates flatten your stomach?

Yes, Pilates can contribute to a flatter stomach. The focus on core engagement in Pilates exercises helps strengthen the deep abdominal muscles, including the transversus abdominis. By consistently practicing Pilates, you can develop a stronger and more toned core, which can lead to a flatter stomach and improved abdominal definition.

4. Is Wall Pilates effective for weight loss?

While Wall Pilates primarily focuses on improving strength, flexibility, and posture, it can indirectly contribute to weight loss. Regular Wall Pilates workouts can increase overall calorie burn, build lean muscle mass, and improve metabolic function. However, for significant weight loss, it is important to combine Wall Pilates with a well-rounded fitness routine that includes cardiovascular exercise and a balanced diet.

5. How do Wall Pilates work for abs?

Wall Pilates can effectively target the abdominal muscles by incorporating exercises that engage the core. Movements such as wall planks, wall sit-ups, and leg lift against the wall can activate the deep abdominal muscles, including the rectus abdominis and obliques. These exercises challenge core stability and strength, leading to improved abdominal tone and strength.

6. What type of Pilates is best for abs?

Traditional Pilates exercises that focus on core engagement, such as Pilates mat exercises, and equipment-based exercises like the Pilates reformer, are effective for strengthening and toning the abs. However, Wall Pilates can also be beneficial for targeting the abdominal muscles, as it offers the added support and resistance of the wall, allowing for deeper engagement and muscle activation.

7. Tips for doing Wall Pilates for abs and glutes

- Maintain proper form and alignment throughout the exercises.
- Engage your core muscles by drawing your navel toward your spine.
- Breathe deeply and rhythmically during each movement.

- Start with exercises that match your fitness level and gradually progress to more challenging variations.
- Incorporate a variety of exercises that target different areas of the abs and glutes.
- Listen to your body and modify or take breaks as needed to avoid overexertion.
- Consistency is key, so aim to practice Wall Pilates for abs and glutes at least 2-3 times a week to see results.

8. When is the right time to start doing Wall Pilates?

Wall Pilates can be suitable for individuals of various ages and fitness levels. However, it is important to consult with a healthcare professional or qualified Pilates instructor if you:

Are over the age of 60 and have not been active for an extended period. Have chronic pain or limited mobility. They can assess your individual needs and provide guidance on how to safely incorporate Wall Pilates into your routine, suggesting modifications or alternative exercises as necessary.

9. What Is Pilates Workout Good For?

Pilates workouts offer numerous benefits, including:

Pilates boosts overall strength and stability by fortifying the deep abdominal and back muscles, resulting in a robust and steadfast core that holds great significance.

Pilates workouts involve movements that stretch and elongate the body, leading to enhanced flexibility, increased joint mobility, and improved muscle elasticity.

10. Is this effective in reducing body fat and toning muscles? Additionally, what is the recommended frequency per week?

Although practicing Wall Pilates may help in shedding weight and shaping the body, it is essential to keep in mind that the attainment of desirable body weight and structure is impacted by a variety of elements such as diet, general physical activity, and genetics. For optimal outcomes, it is advisable to blend Wall Pilates with a comprehensive physical training regimen comprising of cardio workouts, resistance training, and a nutritious diet.

Printed in Great Britain
by Amazon

25908912R00056